CW00449644

The Only Way Is Up

by

Sandi Europe

Realise deeply that the present moment
is all you ever have. Make the Now the
primary focus of your life.
Eckharte Tolle – 'The Power of Now'

Yesterday is history, tomorrow is a
mystery, today is a gift of God which is
why we call it the present.
Bill Keane

Change the way you look at things and
the things you look at will change.
Dr. Wayne W. Dyer

Dedications

There are so many people to whom I owe thanks and gratitude. Primarily this book is for my wonderful sons who make me so proud, André and Richard.

For my grandchildren when they're old enough to read this – Evie, Arianna and Amaiya.

Doctor Ajay Kumar, the miracle worker without whose magic touch my wonderful life would not have been possible.

The amazing staff and nurses from Family Nursing and Home Care who looked after me so well.

My great friend, through good times and bad, Rachel Wilkinson.

For editorial assistance, Roy McCarthy.

There are others who have contributed to my story within these pages, but also countless more people, impossible to list here, who have enhanced my life. You will know who you are, and I thank you so much.

The Spanish Islands

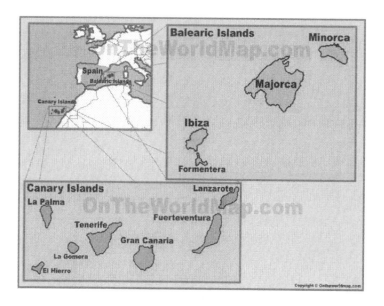

Table of Contents

Objects in the rear-view mirror

It was long ago and it was far away, oh God it seems so very far.
And if life is just a highway, then the soul is just a car
(Jim Steinman)

Looking back, I guess my early years were a bit like Dorothy in Kansas, or Cliff Richard and the Shadows in London. Grey, monochrome. I suppose there must have been colour in there somewhere but I don't recall much. Certainly nothing like the rich palette that I've experienced since.

I was born Sandra Elizabeth Pointing in Altrincham, Cheshire in March 1956. I grew up with my parents (and later, my younger brother and sister) in Sale. It was a nice, respectable area and we owned one of the tidy semi-detached houses that stand along that road.

I wasn't really interested then, but the surname Pointing seems to have first arisen in Devon back in medieval times. My father Derek came from the Birmingham area, but I have no idea what happened in between. My mother Eileen had Irish blood, possibly Romany, and some of what happened to me in later life might be explained in part by some Irish mystical connection.

Post-war rationing had finally ended and Dad was an assistant manager with Barclays Bank, a secure and

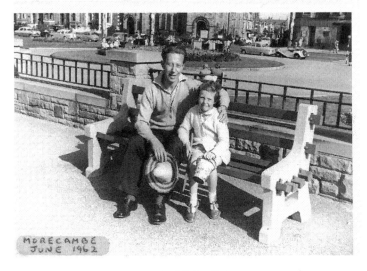

MORECAMBE
JUNE 1962

Dad & Sandi

respectable position. In looks, he might have been the double of Coronation Street's Ken Barlow, and might indeed have been connected in some way to William Roache. He drove a grey/blue Ford Popular. I even remember the number plate – 249 NTU. It must have been his first car and he kept it immaculate. We'd travel in it once a year to Snowdon and Colwyn Bay in North Wales. Lord knows how it always made it there and back. I was really sad when he traded it in for a newer model.

Mum was well-educated and held down a well-paid job in the Civil Service. Mum was quite beautiful and I would always compare her to Elizabeth Taylor. For better or

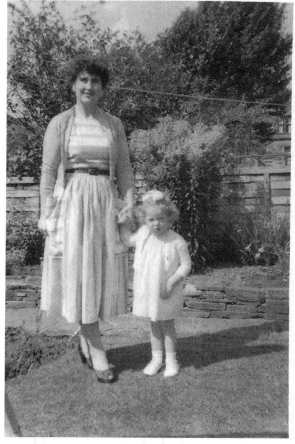

Mum & Sandi

worse, their first child (me) came along. As we know, life is never the same again for a couple after they start a family.

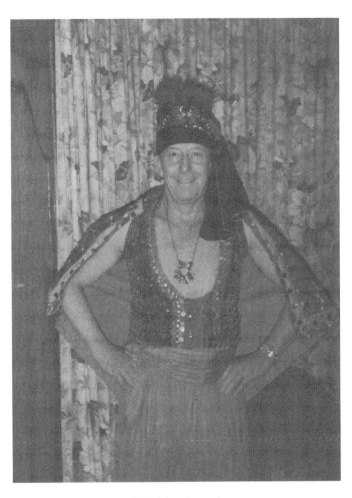

Dad liked dressing up!

My first school was Woodheys Primary, just a short walk away. Most children walked to school in those days, rain or shine. If I tell you that I didn't like school, that would be an understatement. I remember very little of those days

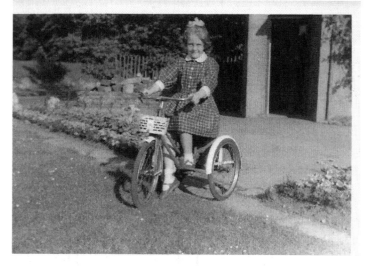

My first bike

– maybe I've sub-consciously blanked them out. I was hopeless at most lessons, couldn't wait for the days to end, my heart sinking at the thought of having to go back the next day. Even at this young age I must have been starting to hope that there was more to life. I don't recall having a favourite teacher, or any particular friends, apart from Allison Holden who has jogged my fading memory. In fact, Allison remembers so much more than I do, so let me hand over to her.

Allison says, 'I first met Sandra at the age of six when my parents moved to Manchester from Carlisle. Sandra and myself were attending the same school, Woodheys Primary School. We went through that school with the same friends -

Susan Marsden, Sylvia Smith, Debra Tomkinson, Julie Holehouse, David Wilkinson, Robert Wood, Howard Pratt. We all then went onto our secondary school, Sale West.

'Sandra and I used to ride our bikes to school every morning and back home for the first few years. Sandra would often stay at my house at a weekend with my Dad making us fried egg sandwiches on a Sunday morning which Sandra loved. I remember going on a school trip to Guernsey and Sandra and I sharing a tent with four other girls.

'We would roll our skirts up so they were shorter once we left the house and met up to go to school. One of the lessons at school that neither of us liked was PE, especially cross country. So what we would do when we were all running was find a shorter route and then end up coming in with the first ones.

'We both started smoking at a young age and used to go around the local shops at lunchtime to have a cigarette. One lunchtime we saw a teacher so both of us ended up putting our cigarettes in our coat pockets and burning a hole.

'We both wore makeup to school and were always getting told off about it. Our school bags in those days were vanity cases so we always made sure we'd get to the back of the classroom so we could lift the lid up and look in the mirror to make sure our mascara and lipstick was OK.

'A few of the male friends I remember were Chris Bartram who possibly was Sandra's first boyfriend, mine *being Gary Oldfield, who sadly passed away at a young age in a motor bike accident. Chris Moran who passed away a few years ago. Gary Kenyon, Brian Bassett, Geoff Langford, Andrew Darbyshire, and we stayed friends with all the girls from Woodheys Primary. When we both left school we went our separate ways but always stayed in contact.*

'Sandra moved to Jersey in 1976 where I joined her in 1978 and lived with her for a few months. I moved back to the UK in 1980.'

At home I don't remember being hugged or loved. I know my father at least was fond of me but, as with most men of the time, he never showed his true feelings. I found a measure of treasured love with my paternal grandmother (my grandfather died when I was five) who lived nearby. I loved going there. There was a big garden with lots of flowers, greenery and a fish pond, with a cricket ground just over the back. I used to sit there for hours. I also remember Nana's neighbours being an Indian family, which was rare in those days as they were very wealthy, living in a large detached house next door. Nana's house was also detached in a very well to do cul-de-sac in Urmston, Manchester. Nana would make me toast with real butter and lime marmalade – what a treat! Mum would cook tripe in milk, which I hated, but I had to eat it or there would be nothing else. I don't think Mum liked cooking very much.

I remember having a wigwam in our garden when I was about eight years old. I loved it and would play in it for hours. Probably, being outdoors, I loved the freedom.

My brother Nigel was born when I was six and my sister Melanie when I was 13. We were never really that close, probably due to such an age gap between the three of us. I sensed my parents were less happy together as the years went by. I believe Mum always regretted the fact that she wasn't able to head off to Australia with her parents and siblings. In those days, if you fitted the criteria, you were able to sail to Australia and start a new life for £10, under the assisted passage scheme. Many thousands did, but Dad resolutely refused to go. For Mum it was a lost opportunity, but what could she do?

As husbands and wives tended to do in those days, they soldiered on. More and more, Dad would take himself away into the 'best room' and work on his stamp collection. He was always on the hunt for rarities, and indeed the pride of his collection was a Penny Black. He would often enjoy listening to jazz. As to parenting, he more or less left Mum to get on with it. We would sit with Mum watching TV, sometimes making toast over the open fire. She loved Dracula and horror films. Her favourite actor was Herbert Lom. On Saturdays we often went to jumble sales as Mum said we couldn't afford new clothes. She would buy us fish and chips, as a treat, on the way home. Looking back, it was strange. Dad was earning well but maybe he was just tight with the housekeeping allowance. In those days, there were many families who were keeping up appearances on a meagre budget.

So mine was a rather dysfunctional family, and became more so. I believe I took my first alcoholic drink when I was 15 on New Year's Eve, looking after my brother and sister when my parents went out. It was Cinzano, which I can't even stand to smell now. I found it took away emotional feelings I didn't then need to deal with. I lived in my head for years rather than my heart.

Eventually Mum and Dad separated, in 1980. It must have been a great release for Dad. He acquired a great interest in Egyptology, travelled to Egypt many times and had a circle of like-minded friends. For Dad it was a new start. He had been in the RAF in his teens and had been to many faraway places, including Egypt, to where he probably wanted to return after the war. But poor Mum. I'd been too young to realise but she started to drink surreptitiously when I was young – 'Sanatogen Wine' she used to wink at me, and I thought it was medicine. It became a more serious problem in years to come, as I was to discover.

I felt alone and left to my own devices, not really having any guidance in my early teens. My mother just seemed to want me to have a boyfriend, then to settle down and get married. I think she thought I needed a man to make me happy as opposed to being single and my own person. I wish I'd had more support to understand what life was all about.

Despite what Allison remembers above, my first boyfriend was Terry. He gave me driving lessons in his Ford Zodiac (the model with the big wings and bench seats). He had a boat moored in Conwy in North Wales. We would go there at weekends, maybe do a bit of boat painting.

By this time, I'd left Woodheys and I'd started at Sale West secondary school (long since closed). I'm afraid my academic performance didn't improve and I continued to bump along hopelessly, trying to see ahead to the day when I'd be able to leave and see what else the world had to offer. At least I had an opportunity to try sports and activities, and I was very good at English which was to help enormously in later years. I went to dancing school, played tennis, tried swimming. At last I found something that appealed to me. At the Cadman School of Dancing I excelled at Latin and danced at the famous Tower Ballroom in Blackpool. Had I only continued, but I was at an age where partying took precedence.

I played tennis at weekends which I really enjoyed. My Dad bought me a bike one Christmas with a gear stick on the lower bar. It was expensive, and very different to my friends' bikes.

And at the tender age of 15 I was suddenly free with not a qualification to my name. I suppose my teachers must have tried their best with me but they were disappointed. So, what to do? I had seen little of life outside Sale and the Manchester area. I needed to get a job. I wanted to train as a hairdresser but Mum said – quite rightly – that there was more money in secretarial work. I found a trainee secretary's position with Anderson's Roofing at Trafford Park, a large industrial estate in Manchester. They sent me to college on day release, and slowly I began to build a skill set which served me well in years to come. There were, however, one or two teeny mistakes. For example, I became a legend there by filling out a chitty directing a driver to Coventry instead of Daventry! They were only 20 miles apart – I don't know why they got so cross.

From Anderson's I moved to another company at Trafford Park, Containerbase, which only served to tantalise me more about the world outside of Manchester. My life still lacked colour. Surely there was more to it than working in an industrial park and living in the Manchester suburbs?

At about age 17 I had a boyfriend, Derek, who lived in Urmston near Nana. I started going on holiday with him, including Amsterdam and Benidorm. I loved Amsterdam and the barges on the river, but Benidorm was just all expats partying. I was later to discover a much different side to Spain.

The Great Escape

I fly through the air with the greatest of ease
Out of the window, over the trees
(Ian Hunter)

It was early 1976 and I was 19. More than ever I was eager to escape the greyness of north-west England. I wasn't unhappy, no bad experiences, nothing like that. I just needed to be free, explore my potential, see different places and experience new things.

To do this I needed money. My parents weren't going to pay for me to scoot off and enjoy myself. I would need to pay my own way. I was willing to do so. I understood from a young age that if I wanted anything more than the bare necessities in life then I was going to have to work for them.

Me and my friend Jackie started writing letters; remember this was before the advent of the internet, e-mail and instant communication. Longhand letters, stick on a stamp, send it off. We wanted a bit of fun as well as work. We wrote many letters and one day we had a reply. It was from Peter Horne of the Seymour Hotel Group in Jersey. I was offered a job for the summer season at Le Coie Hotel, in St Helier! 'Supervisor of Chambermaids.' Never mind that I had never done this before. It was a classic case of 'land the job, then learn how to do it'. Jackie was also offered a job at the same hotel. Preparations made, notices handed in, we were on our way with great excitement and expectations.

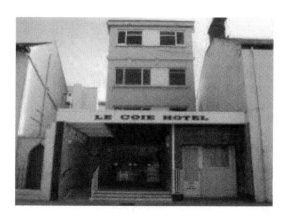

Le Coie Hotel, long gone.

We flew down to Jersey from Manchester Airport in March and found our way to Le Coie. At that time the Jersey tourism scene was at its height and Le Coie Hotel was one of the largest hotels on the island with some 300 bedrooms. It was on the outskirts of St Helier and therefore handy for the busy shops and vibrant pub and nightclub scene. (Le Coie closed in the 1990s, along with many others, as tourism declined. The site is now apartments.)

Jersey in 1976 was all that I'd hoped for and imagined. That year was one of the hottest and driest on record, and of course it was the same for the UK generally. The 'greyness' of Manchester – real or imagined – was gone. From the moment we landed in Jersey everything was bright and cheerful. Even though I was working a 6-day week, it felt as if I, too, were on holiday. At least to begin with.

Jackie quickly became homesick and went home, but I'd already started making new friends. I met and shared a room with a girl called Terri. At weekends there were the fabulous beaches and by night there was a non-stop partying scene. Those were the halcyon days for tourism. Jersey's most famous beach is St Brelade's Bay and the crowds would flock there. It was my favourite and, naively (though in common with many others) got sunburnt too often until I learnt sense and understood that my pale skin was an easy target for the hot Jersey sun if left uncovered. In fact, I contracted skin cancer at one stage and had a lesion cut out. They were the days of ignorance as regards skin cancer and goodness knows how many others suffered as we had no knowledge that such danger existed. Similar skin problems were to vex me for years to come.

Terri says, 'I first met Sandra back in March 1976. The long, hot summer I'll never forget. I was working in London in a hotel on the Strand as a hotel housekeeper in charge of ten ladies. I'd attended hotel and catering college and was on a path to be a hotel manager.

'I arrived in Jersey on the 19th March, Sandra's birthday, in a snow storm. I was welcomed at the hotel and shown my accommodation. The house was next door to the hotel and I was told I was sharing it with the two other housekeepers who were due to arrive later in the week. My heart sank. It was freezing and damp and we were given two connecting rooms.

'I started work the next day and was greeted by the head housekeeper Mrs Therin, a force to be reckoned with! I was

informed Sandra and Edwina were due later – neither had previous experience of hotel work. Naturally, someone with college and London experience was rather surprised to hear this and wondered what pleasures were in store. Sandra arrived smiling, her bubbly self and pleasant personality shone through.

'Rotas were put together and over the next month we all got along and adjusted to life in a seasonal holiday hotel, massively different to what I was used to.'

The sea sports crowd would frequent the wide sweep of St Ouen's Bay on the west coast, or perhaps Plemont in the north with its caves and lively swell. The coastal roads of the island were nose to tail with hire cars, and with coaches (anti-clockwise in the morning, clockwise in the afternoon) seeking out the smaller bays, the many attractions and the tea rooms and cafés that catered for the holidaymakers. Dads eyed the country pubs thirstily.

Terri says,' The weather however wasn't good, at least not at first. It was cold and wet. The town was dreary and we were fed up of the local pubs and night life. The town seemed to be rather dated and we needed fun. I also was extremely ill with a kidney infection due to the damp room and bed. Poor Edwina had had enough and went back to the mainland.

'The doctor insisted the management moved Sandra and I out of the rooms. We were told we had to share the front bedroom or move to the other side of town! I had never

shared a room but as I am an only child, I thought this may be fun!

'I'll never forget that first night Sandra came in the worse for wear in the small hours, switched on the light, then fell over the one-bar electric fire. I was not impressed and the language was colourful.'

In the evenings the older holidaymakers would head for one of the many shows and cabarets on offer. Coach ride, show ticket, scampi-in-the-basket all in the price. There was Caesar's Palace, New Mediterranean, Swanson's, the Hawaiian at Portelet, Behan's, Birdcage etc. By day, Leah Bell and Johnny de Little would sing at the Fort and by night do the night club circuit. Famous UK acts were plentiful with Dustin Gee and Les Dennis, and the Krankies, being typical and popular acts. Dancing girls were a staple of any show and a handy way of earning a few quid in the summer if you could high-kick in rhythm.

Us younger ones preferred the pubs and the clubs. Booze and fags were amazingly cheap in the 1970s and did we take advantage. The Top Hat, Kon Tiki, Blue Fox, Les Arches, Skyline, Lords, Adrian's, Watersplash, many more. These were the places where the partying took place, the drink flowed and the music played till late. Dare I say it was where boy met girl and many affairs, often fleeting, occasionally longer lasting, began under the glittering lights of Jersey's discos and night clubs. I wasn't immune, I must confess.

Terri says, 'We had been on the Island just over a month and had Saturday nights off together (good roster planning). We soon learned that Les Arches night club out at Archirondel was the place to be. We were on a mission.

'Our mission paid off and we arrived back home in a car accompanied by Mark and Allan. Fortunately, the boys were good friends and we all spent time together exploring the Island. By the end of April the sun had come out and the fun started. Oh, and we worked our socks off too. We were effectively thrown together and under any other circumstances would not have met. I'm so pleased we did. I learned that Sandra was a very good secretary. She had a lovely way with the staff and I discovered a very different approach that was not taught at college. She even tried to learn Portuguese!'

October came and the hotel was closing for the winter. What was I to do? I was desperate not to have to return back to Manchester having tasted freedom. I looked around – fortunately I'd had a certain amount of secretarial experience which I could offer prospective employers. In the meantime, Le Coie kindly let me continue to live in their staff flats. I landed my first office job in Jersey. It was at the offices of Coopers & Lybrand, Chartered Accountants, in La Motte Street. In fact I took over the job from Joyce, a woman who became, and remains, a great friend.

Joyce says 'I came to Jersey with my family and we made our home there. Dad was a bit of an entrepreneur and he bought a guest house in Clarendon Road, a garage, a boarding house. He even considered buying what was to become the Hotel L'Emeraude. Sadly Dad died and Mum sold the businesses, and I continued to live with her.

'In the late 1970s I worked for Abacus Trust, at that time a small part of the much larger Coopers & Lybrand. There were about 100 staff in all at that time. That's where I first met Sandra. Along with many others from the firm we used to frequent the Lillie Langtry bar, just over the road. They used to do fabulous lunches for 50p.'

As luck would have it, a client of the firm owned a house at Mont Mado, St John, with a flat attached, and this became my next home. It was a lovely old granite farmhouse, typical 'Jersey', with an annexe.

In those days the local 'scene' for many during the winter was the Rugby Club. Before the present impressive building went up, the changing rooms and bar were in a single, long building situated where the car park now is. The place was legendary, especially on weekend evenings. Visiting teams were entertained there and the booze flowed. And somehow people contrived to drive home. It was there that I met a new boyfriend, Alan, a rugby player. Followed by Bill, an American printer, with whom I lived in a bedsit at First Tower for a short time, next to the former First Tower Inn, another pub long closed and forgotten. Bill's mother was a GI bride.

We were both happy at first, but Bill became fed up in Jersey. He wanted to find a printing job in the hot sunshine far away. I wrote professional-type letters to places in Saudi using my secretarial skills, and Bill was offered a printing job. I assumed he'd come back – Saudi wasn't somewhere that I particularly wanted to go to. He never came back. He stayed for a few years then returned to the USA, married an American girl and had more children. I found this out many years later when I became curious; he already had a daughter from a previous relationship in the UK.

A few years ago, when I was in Spain, I went to see a clairvoyant. She saw Bill clearly, described him exactly. That meant only one thing to me. Sure enough, I searched for, and found, his obituary notice. He died only aged 68.

So my new life progressed. I had a variety of jobs after Coopers, amongst them being estate agents Viberts, Troys, Gothard & Trevor, builders' merchants Huelins, Randalls Brewery, and also Mourants lawyers in Hill Street.

The nicest job I had was with Trafalgar House Investments, Hope Street, who were then a small cog in Jersey's burgeoning finance industry. Keith Lawrence was a great boss. I paid the staff on cruise ships. I had the opportunity of going cruising for free, but never took up the opportunity. Maybe I thought cruising was just for the elderly. I wouldn't hesitate today. I love cruising, waking up in a new place every day. I was to do several cruises in the years to come.

Love and Marriage

I met Richard Tanguy (Dick), a lorry driver, whilst working a couple of evenings a week at St Mary's Country Hotel. One evening we went to a party in Roseville Street together. He threw a tomato at me. He was smoking pot and I flushed his joint down the toilet. (I believe that this was the same party where a jealous woman threatened Joyce with a knife, but the incident was defused.) We decided to get married, and therein lies a tale, and it involves us getting married not once but twice. After only a short while together we booked the church with the Reverend Peter Manton. We had our eyes on a property in Poonah Lane, St Helier to be our marital home. However, we needed a States Loan, which used to be available to those starting out on the property ladder. The horrible woman at the Housing Department snorted that, in order to qualify, we needed to be married. It was no good that we were at the planning stage. We explained this to Rev. Manton. 'No problem,' he said, 'you can be legally married straightaway and then proceed with the church wedding in due course.' So that's exactly what happened. We married secretly in June 1979 and went ahead with the 'real' wedding in the August, both at St John's Church. Happily, my family were all in Jersey to attend the 'real' wedding.

Allison and her boyfriend were at the 'secret' wedding. Allison was dating Dick's best friend Rod Le Cornu and they were to marry, but then also divorce.

We honeymooned in Greece, travelling first to Athens, then the Greek islands. It was so hot.

Joyce says 'Sandra and I were both newly married, but we still decided to head off on holiday together. We went to Cannes, and had a fun time. We were still young and naïve in many respects and we raised our eyebrows at things like topless sunbathing, the proliferation of strange night clubs and so on. At one stage we ended up, the pair of us, riding along the seafront behind some bloke on a motor bike, no helmets of course.'

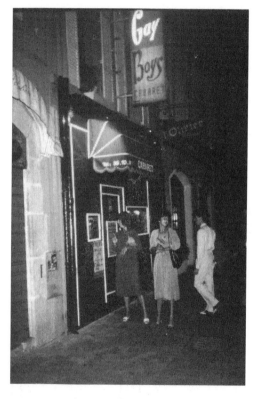

Gay Boys Cabaret, Cannes

'We took a train up to Monte Carlo and visited a casino. With limited funds we just drank tap water and *watched the proceedings, fascinated by the rich old women draped in gold, swanning around the place. Then we somehow missed our train station and ended up across the Italian border in Sanremo. There were no trains back that evening so we had to stay the night. That was ok as I enjoyed eating proper Italian food for the first time! Happy days.'*

Meanwhile my mother and father had separated. He had become more withdrawn and fascinated by Egypt and his collection of Egyptology. My mother dedicated herself more and more to the bottle. She, together with Nigel and Melanie, came to live with us in Jersey for a while after we married. We had bought the little house in Poonah Lane, in town. Hosting the family was a mistake and a nightmare. Mum was drinking heavily – we hadn't realised how bad she had become. We would find bottles hidden all over the house. She had ceased to care about her appearance and she was very argumentative. Had I known about Alcoholics Anonymous then, it might have been an answer. As it was though I nearly had a breakdown trying to cope with her.

Dick had had enough, finding bottles all over the house which Mum had tried to hide. Dick used to make his own beer and she would drink it, and the dregs. Very sad. I saw a woman of standing turn into someone who I didn't recognise at all, someone who just didn't care about herself. I went to the Samaritans for help, but to little avail. Dick said, 'She goes or I go!'

Mum eventually returned to the UK leaving her children behind. We looked after them as best we could. I hoped that Dad might have helped at this time, but perhaps he had his own issues. Nigel went to Highlands College to study catering while Melanie attended Les Quennevais School. After a while they both moved back to the UK to live with our father.

However, Melanie did enjoy her time in Jersey and she eventually came back. Back in Manchester she'd met a guy called Steve. By then Dick and I had bought a large house in St Lawrence but there was an economic slump in the 80s and we were having difficulty affording the mortgage payments without taking in students and lodgers. We converted the garage and Melanie and Steve came to live there until they found their own flat.

Our eldest boy, André was born in 1984, and Richard in 1986. I was fully expecting girls and had bought girls' clothing, but I wouldn't trade either for the world. We all travelled to Disneyworld once the boys were old enough. From when they were eight/six years old we'd regularly go to Club La Santa in Lanzarote. It was (and still is) a sporting Mecca and the boys were in their element. Many top athletes would use the place for warm weather training and, amongst others, we were lucky enough to meet the boxer Frank Bruno and Olympic javelin silver medallist Steve Backley. It wasn't all fun though. Richard was running around one day and fell into a garden of cacti. He was in a lot of pain with the spines cutting into his hands and arms.

We eventually got them all out but he was certainly in

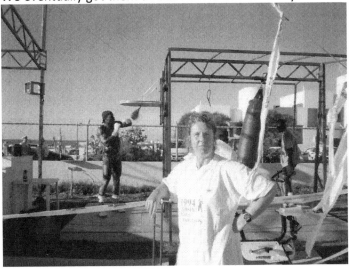

Club La Santa with Frank Bruno

shock, my poor little one, but no hospital necessary on this occasion.

André says 'I attended Bel Royal School and Les Quennevais before transferring to Hautlieu. I was always sporty – I played footy a lot. I guess running/cross country and athletics was my 'thing'. I was with Jersey Spartans for several years in the 1990s, running track but also learning and competing in various field events. A bit of cycling too. At Bournemouth university I studied sports science and TV production, but spent much of my time surfing.'

Richard says 'My first primary school was St Lawrence, then when we moved into town, I attended Bel

Royal School. I then moved up to Les Quennevais School. As now, I enjoyed most sports – badminton, soccer, hockey, karate, though I wasn't particularly outstanding at them. I learnt swimming and diving at Jersey Swimming Club under Roy Horsfall and John Fage. I turned to cycling, and later triathlon, a little more successfully. Biology was my favourite academic subject. I moved on to Hautlieu before heading off to Exeter University to study Sports and Exercise Science.'

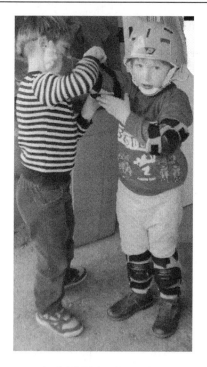

André & Richard

In my early years of marriage, I worked at the Jersey Evening Post at Five Oaks in the advertising section. It was the time that Frank Walker, a future Chief Minister, was Chairman there. Peter Tabb was my first boss followed by David Edwards, and I got on well with the late Christine Morgan. (Sadly and oddly, Christine died due to an abscess on her gum at about the same time my youngest son Richard was born, and he has an almost identical personality to her.) I also worked for a time as PA to the accountant Leonard Day. I also part-owned Fleur-de-Lys, a florists' wholesalers, in Commercial Street for a time.

But sadly, our marriage was not to last. In my view (though not Dick's) it had run its course. We separated in 2000, and were divorced in 2007. I regarded our parting as a second chance, and I hold Dick totally blameless in this. Little did I know what I was to achieve on my own.

Running

Rewinding a few years now, to about 1994, I'd started doing a little bit of running with Jersey Spartan Athletics Club, and later, the Crapaud Hash House Harriers. With the competitive Spartans I was among the slower runners and it was there, towards the back of the pack, I met Rachel Wilkinson. Rachel was to become not only a great running and rowing partner, but a great friend. She also has a much better memory of those times so here I'll hand over to Rachel.

Rachel says, 'At the time my two boys were getting bigger and I decided to take up a bit of running again, with Daphne Wagstaffe at Spartans. (Daphne was to be tragically killed a few years later.) I got chatting to Sandra as one does in social running situations. We are both 1956-born and we decided to enter the 1996 London Marathon for our 40th birthdays, raising money in the process for the Variety Club. I'm not quite sure how, but we both managed to succeed in the entry ballot. Our entries were accepted and we supposed we had better start training rather more seriously.

'In those days Spartans used to hold a series of races designed to lead up to Spring marathons, still a popular thing to do among Club members at the time. We ran these and were confident as we travelled to London the night before and got stuck in at the pasta party.

'The great day dawned, and it dawned very warmly. The temperature was to rise to about 30 degrees during the day. I remember well the rhino-heads who were competing, and the man with the ladder (for conquering the dreaded Wall). At some stage I pulled away from Sandra. They ran out of water at some stage and we were offered refills from dustbins full of greasy liquid – I declined. I ran and chatted with a 74-year old bloke at one stage but shamefully was determined to beat him.

'I finished in an official time of 5:21.53. Sandra was not so far behind, happily jogging in to record 5:41.35.

'We continued running for a time afterwards with the likes of Christine Ritchie, Sheila Le Boutillier, Sue Furnival and Shirley Rowe until we discovered another interest.'

It was through running that I met a lifelong friend Dawn Wheeler. Originally from Plymouth, she had also arrived in Jersey via Guernsey in 1976.

> *Dawn says, 'When I arrived in Jersey I worked at the old Grève d'Azette Hotel. In those days that area was buzzing and lively with all the bars and nightspots. It's all apartments now. I went on to work in hospitality, owning the Old Station Café at Millbrook at one time, and an ice-cream business, the café at Ouaisné.*
>
> *'I met Sandi one day when we were with the Crapaud Hash House Harriers. God knows what I was doing there because I was never a runner. I think it was some sort of relay and I'd been roped in to make up the numbers. We lost contact for a while after that.'*

Rowing

Yes, it was me that introduced Rachel to rowing, but I'm so glad we had those days. Running along Jersey's cliff paths I used to get glimpses of rowing boats in the sea down below and thought it looked fun. So it came to pass that we bought a boat, four of us. There was a Finnish girl, Maggie Tornoroth in bow, I was no.2, Rachel was no.3 and Jean Bertram was stroke. Again, I'll hand over to Rachel.

> *Rachel says 'We named our boat Maid Tuin and joined the Jersey Rowing Club. Training in the winter (which no one else seemed to do) we persuaded one or two experienced people to take us out and show us the ropes. We got the hang of it with the result that, when the Spring races re-started, we did very well and put a few noses out of joint.*

We were total novices but we had a great time and a great laugh. Sandra always seemed to need a pee just before the start of a race and the bailer had to be deployed to our great merriment and the disdain of other crews.

'We had some success in the local races, and entered the Sark – Jersey race on three occasions, winning our class. We set what I believe may still be a fixed-seat record in the Round-the-Island race. We also took part in the Gorey-Carteret race, and also in the subsequent party antics.

'Another memorable race was a London river race where, to comply with the rules, we had to carry a passenger. This turned out to be the reluctant 15-year old son of the Mayor of Tower Hamlets and he turned out to be a liability in the first degree.

'Life eventually got in the way and the girls went their separate ways. Maid Tuin was sold, though it is still being used to this day. Sandra and I thought it was a good idea to buy a 2-man boat called Top Banana. Sculling proved beyond us however and we eventually sold this boat as well. Days never to be forgotten.'

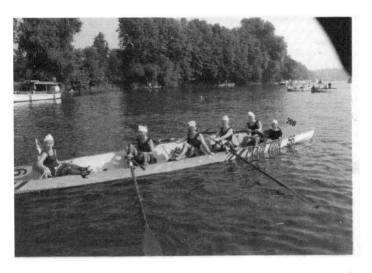

On the Thames - Alison, Jean, Rachel, Sandi, Maggie & Vicky

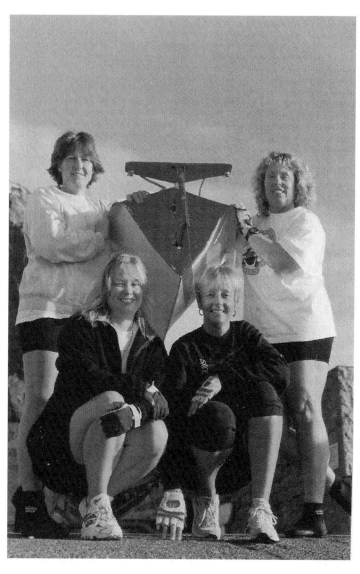

Rachel, Maggie, Jean, Sandi

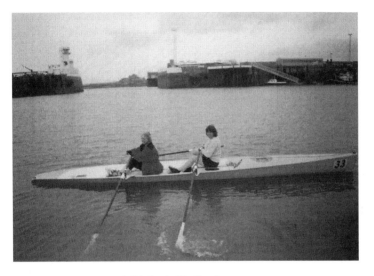

With Rachel in Top Banana

Then it All Stopped

I wondered why my circumstance
had turned out as it had
What had I done to cause
a situation quite this bad
(Cheryl Davis Miller)

After my separation from Dick I bought an old Victorian flat on two floors in Mont Cochon at First Tower – this was in 2000 when André was 15 and Richard was 13. I was living on my own with the boys. The flat was perfect as the upper floor was in the attic with two bedrooms. The boys would spend much time up there with their friends, probably smoking pot and drinking. It was their hideaway and they could play loud music without getting told off. Well, sometimes I would say something but I think I gave them a lot of leeway, more than I ever had as a teenager.

I hadn't though reckoned on having the Neighbours From Hell.

However, I spent much of this time travelling, enjoying myself. André soon finished school and went off to Bournemouth University. Richard would stay with his Dad when I went away. I took in a lodger, George, and he became a good friend. He was my companion on a couple of cruises. We went to stay at my father's cousin's house in Maine Island, off Vancouver Island in Canada. Before that, also with George, I went on a real cheapie cruise from Genoa around the Mediterranean islands. It was my first cruise and the ship was old and there was no water in the

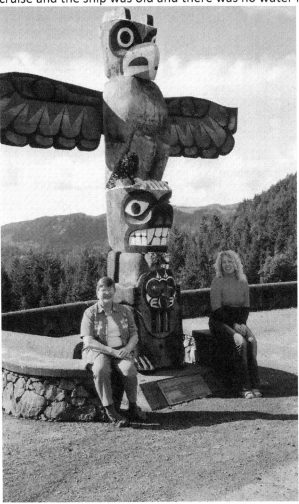

Vancouver Island with Dad's cousin Janet

swimming pool. We did meet some interesting people and (as usual for me) I met a clairvoyant from Italy. She wanted to speak with me. She read my cards and said I had neighbours at home who were colluding against me. This later proved to be the case.

Other trips included Thailand with my rowing buddy Jean Bertram, also South Africa with my close friend Maggie Begeman, who sadly died a few years ago. We met through our children. My eldest, André, was friends with her son Andy. We travelled often together – South Africa, France, other places that I can't immediately recall. Maggie was a carer at St Saviour's Hospital here in Jersey. She often complained of a bad back, but assumed it was the occupational hazard of lifting patients. Eventually she got it checked out. It was incurable cancer of the spine. I returned from Spain to be with her for a while. Sadly, the cancer spread quickly and Maggie died in August 2014. I still miss her and wish I could have had one last chat with her.

Australia

Australia in November 2004 was a great highlight for me. Richard was selected for the Jersey cycling team to compete at the Commonwealth Youth Games in Bendigo, Victoria, best known for its days as a gold rush town. Richard had always been sporty, as you'll have noted previously.

Others on the Jersey team which travelled to Australia were Jersey Spartan athletes Lauren Therin and Stephen Prosser. Poor Stephen, a talented sprinter, crashed out in his 100-metre heat when leading, with a knee injury which ended his career in the sport. Lauren however picked

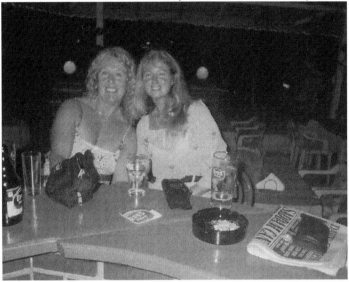

With Maggie Begeman

up bronze medals in javelin and discus. Richard competed well to finish 9th in the road race and 11th in the time trial.

> Richard says, 'The Commonwealth Youth Games is up there as perhaps the sporting highlight of my young life. It was a fantastic and unexpected opportunity. Dad travelled with the Jersey team as my sort-of chaperone/team manager. We stopped off in Singapore en route for a few days' preparation before going on to Melbourne and then Bendigo where the Games were held.
>
> 'The trip was fun, and there was a good team spirit. As to training, I was still pretty young and inexperienced. I

just did what I was told without knowing too much about the science behind it.

'I had a blast in the road race. I found myself in a breakaway group with the likes of Ian Stannard, Ben Swift and Matt Goss, all of whom went on to become professional cyclists. I was delighted to finish in the top ten in that company. By contrast, the time trial was an anti-climax, though I didn't do too bad I suppose.

'Mum came out and I met her there, but we were quickly on the way home once the Games ended. Mum was to stay on and see long-lost family.'

Beyond this, it was a great opportunity for me to visit family in Melbourne and Brisbane. I stayed with my Mum's brother and his family. It was great to eventually meet my cousins. I went to Brisbane to visit my Dad's cousin. She was in her 80s but still partying! My uncle Ian (Mum's brother) also had a house in Cairns and I accepted his offer to stay there for a few days. I took the opportunity to visit Hamilton Island close to the Great Barrier Reef, with my cousin Nick. What an amazing place.

And then

The years 2000 – 2004 after my separation were, in one sense, halcyon years. I had my freedom, my travelling which I loved, my wonderful growing sons. If it hadn't been for the Neighbours From Hell then perhaps my life would have continued on much the same course. The NFH had no intention of co-existing peacefully, least of all with any measure of friendliness. Where I come from, neighbours might have bickered at times but they were always there to lend a hand if you needed one and would always stop for a friendly chat. Not these two.

From the outset there were confrontations about parking, rights and obligations, etc. They considered that I should remove the old, original outside steps that led up to my front door as something that would help solve the problem – their perceived problem, not mine. In other small ways they were intimidating. It got to the stage where I felt their eyes boring into me if I left the house. I was on my own with the boys, often only Richard. I felt alone, isolated and nervous. I started, like my poor mother, drinking a little too much. I'd either go out and drink for the companionship, or maybe I'd have an unnecessary glass or two too much at home.

Was this a contributory factor in what happened that night? Yes, undoubtedly. But what happened next changed my life for ever.

I'd been out with a friend – let's call him Simon. We'd met online and I hadn't known him long. My friends didn't like him, they thought he was hiding something. We'd had drinks at the Grand Hotel, and I'd naturally had plenty of them. We got a taxi home and I let us both into the house. I remember going upstairs to check that Richard was in. The next thing I recall is that I was at the bottom of the stairs. I'd somehow slipped and fallen. I tried to get up, but I couldn't move. I felt my neck crack, I couldn't push with my arms. I knew it was serious. Though that night is a blur, I do remember Simon being there when I fell. He just vanished, left me for dead. Why didn't he call an ambulance?

I called out to Richard, but it was a weak effort and he was fast asleep. Time and again I called, and maybe two hours later he heard me. He called for an ambulance. And as they loaded me into the ambulance, I swear I saw the NFH at the window, looking at me expressionless.

Richard says, 'I awoke to someone screaming and shouting my name. I found Mum lying at the bottom of the stairs.
'Mum, are you all right? Come on get up into bed.'
'I can't.'
'Get up, don't be stupid.'
'I can't get up.' I went and got a duvet and put it over her.
'Mum, in five minutes I'll call an ambulance if you're still there.'
'OK, give me five minutes.' Five minutes went by.
'You have to get up now Mum, please.'
'I can't get up.'

'The ambulance arrived. They tried to move Mum but she screamed the place down. They tried to put her into a chair, then used the spinal board. They took us both to the General Hospital. I spent the night there.

'It's surreal, looking back. Like watching an old film. I was only 17 and just dealt as best I could with what was in front of me at the time.'

Coming To

The sun will come out
Nothing good ever comes easy
(Kali Uchis)

28th February 2005, morning

White squares swim into my vision. I blink a few times, trying to focus, but everything remains blurry. I am perplexed. What are these lines and shapes on the ceiling? They should not be there. Something about them is wrong.

Although my eyes have only been open for a few moments, I feel tired from looking at the strange shapes above me, trying to work them out. There is an uncomfortable feeling in my shoulders, and my arms feel constricted, tense. Pain everywhere in my upper body. I want to roll over onto my side, find a better position. I attempt to shift around. After a few moments of struggle, I find that I cannot move at all. In the end I give up and lie there, panting from the exertion. My bewilderment and confusion grow.

Sometime later I open my eyes again – I must have drifted off. My head feels fuzzy and heavy. There is pressure behind my eyes and I can hear blood rushing in my ears. My neck and shoulders are really sore, like I have been sleeping in the same position all night. A throbbing sensation between my shoulder blades. My eyes readjust to the luminosity of the room. The square shapes in the ceiling above me begin to converge again – I remember them from before. What is this? Have the boys done something in my bedroom? I squint. Something about these squares disturb me. Then I notice the sound of the alarm clock. It seems to be stuck, slowly beeping away by my side. I must turn it off and get up. God knows what time it is.

I try and fail to lift my head off the pillow. Agitation sets in. What is wrong? I have to get up! Why am I so weak? I muster all my energy to lift my upper body. Nothing happens, nothing at all. My limbs seem dead. I feel so tired. What did I do last night? I can't remember.

I try to gather my thoughts. Something on the edge of my consciousness is bothering me. There is something I need to remember. Something bad. What is it? I struggle to think but I'm at a loss. I must call Richard. 'Richard?' My voice comes out as a hoarse whisper. I try to wet my lips with a dry tongue and try again. 'Richard?' Nothing. He must have gone to school. Is it Monday?

I listen to the slow beeping of the alarm clock. Wait. That sound isn't right. Has someone changed the sound? 'Richard?' I try again, louder. No one comes. I begin to feel frightened. Have I had a stroke or something? Richard is out, there's no one to help me. My head pounds and my vision clouds over.

I blink a few times, trying to revive my sore, prickly eyes. The square shapes in the ceiling come into focus again. I frown. They look like...tiles? Big, white industrial ceiling tiles. This is strange, my bedroom doesn't have ceiling tiles. Finally, it occurs to me that this may not be my bedroom. Can I be in Maggie's bedroom? Relief pours over me. Of course. I must have stayed over at Maggie's place. I'm not going mad after all, thank God! I'm somewhere else, not in my own bedroom. The relief is immense. 'Maggie?' Finally! I hear the bedroom door open, footsteps approaching, a smiling face above me. But it's not Maggie.

'OK there Sandra? Awake? Good.' The smiling woman disappears, but I can hear her there, doing something nearby. It sounds as if she's opening a plastic wrapper. I fight the thick haze that envelopes me, desperate to understand. What is going on? My heart beat rises in strength and speed along with my anxiety levels. The alarm clock beeps on. Then I notice for the first time a faint sterile, antiseptic smell. 'Oh, this is....' I think, 'This is...oh my God!'

28th February 2005, midday

Oh no, oh no, oh no this can't be happening. What have I done to myself?

I lie there, looking up, unable to shift even a finger. I am stuck, trapped, as good as dead. This cannot be happening...but it is. You see these scenes on the telly, Saturday night, other people's lives, but it's real, there's nothing I can do. What have you done Sandra?

I think feverishly, in desperation. If only I could rewind the tape, go back to whatever moment this began. I fell, I think. The stairs. Just let me be at the top of the stairs again, start again from there. Stop this horror from unfolding.

Stupid, stupid, stupid woman. I have been a brainless person, living wrong, irresponsibly, doing stupid things. This is the result. My punishment. I would do anything now to be saved. Change my ways, be different.

Oh God, please, I really need you now. I will do anything if you just make this go away. Please God, please. This is surreal, need to pinch myself.

28th February 2005, afternoon

'Hello Sandra, are we awake?'

Startled, I open my eyes. I have been lost in thought. The kind, young face I saw earlier is back again. She is pretty, her plump apple cheeks framed with blond hair. I take in the blue uniform and two blue eyes lined with heavy black eye liner which smile at me. 'Just here to change the drip, won't take long, try to rest.' I try to say something to her, but my throat will not work. I open and close my mouth like a fish

'Good. Very good.' She is stretching her vowels in an attempt to sound comforting. 'Now, try not to worry. The doctor will come along soon and this afternoon we will be taking you for some X-rays. We can see about a drink later, ok?'

Do I have a choice?

'There. The doctor won't be long now. Try to rest.' In a flurry of efficient footsteps, she is gone. A door opens somewhere to my far left, bringing a brief gush of cooler air and the sound of people talking. Then it swooshes shut. I am left on my own, and I experience a pang, a small, jagged feeling of desperation in the centre of my chest. My life has boiled down to this.

I am stuck here, just me and my thoughts. Clenching my jaw, I try not to think about the future lest my quiet desperation grow into panic.

2nd March 2005, afternoon

'Hi Mum, how's it going?' I hear footsteps, then Richard is standing over me. My heart flips when I see the look on his face. He looks so tall, but still so young.
'OK, considering,' I croak. 'How was school?'
'Oh good. Yeah, school's all right.' He seems pleased about my answer, and glad to change the subject away from me. 'We had PE, played football. Oh wait.' He moves away and I can hear him walking around the bed. He reappears on the other side. 'The nurse is here Mum.'
Another face appears; it is the male nurse this time, older than the young girls who usually come. 'Hello there, Sandra. Got your son visiting you today!' The nurse checks the drip with deft hands.
'Yes, it's nice to see him.' I try to sound as cheery as he does.
'Any problems? Nausea? Pain? Headache?'
'Umm, some pain in my neck. No headache. No sickness.'
'OK, I'll make a note. We'll see if the doctor can up the pain killers a little bit this evening.' He scratches notes onto his clipboard, gives the drip tube a tap, then moves along to the next bed. 'Bye for now.'

Richard and I are left to ourselves. 'So, did the doctor come, Mum?'
'Yes, the doctor was here. They're going to operate as soon as possible. They are going to put a titanium plate in my

neck. I'll be like the Bionic Lady.'
'It's Bionic Woman, Mum.'
'Oh,' I say. 'Well I do beg your pardon – Bionic Woman then. I'll probably bleep when I go through airport security.'
We both giggle. 'Doctor Kumar says that I'm lucky to be alive. I was half a centimetre from severing my spinal cord.'
Richard was silent.

> Richard says, 'I visited my Mum a number of times in hospital. I think the first time I was fully aware of the seriousness of the matter was when I saw her in her halo neck brace. I think I knew then that hard times lay ahead, but, at that age, I didn't really have the knowledge to understand or process the possible implications.'

Then his face turns serious again and the child is back. 'So, does that mean...'? He pauses, unsure how to finish the sentence, but I can easily guess.
'Well, Doctor Kumar seems positive. I mean, I might have to be in a wheelchair for a while, just at first, but I think it'll be all fine in the end, with physio and so on. I might need some help from you in the beginning though, but I'm sure it won't be for long.'
Richard nods, taking it all in, processing the news. If I could then I would squeeze his hand right now. 'Honestly Richard, you don't need to worry about me. I'll be fine, you'll see. I'll be back at home driving you mad again soon.' I'm not sure if Richard believes me. He puts on a polite smile, but he looks down and fiddles with the edge of my pillow. I don't know what to say any more, so I change the subject. 'Can you do me a favour before you go? Just put those flowers in some

water into that vase? The nurse was going to do it but she got called away, shame if they were to wilt.'

Looking relieved to have something to do, Richard sets off to the ward kitchen and I listen to his trainers squeaking down the corridor

This isn't bloody fair. He is too young to be nursing a mother in a wheelchair and helping with bedpans. I am still young too. I'm not ready to give up so much of my life yet. I have so much I want to do. Since my separation five years ago I have not stopped travelling – South Africa, Las Vegas, France, Thailand, Canada, Spain. Maggie and I had been planning the USA next, and there are so many other places I haven't been to yet, and what about…? Here my courage falters. I cannot think about a life with no dating, no men, no sex. No more chance to love a man. It's not fair. I think I deserve another opportunity to be happy? Don't I?

'Mum?' Richard comes back, filled vase in hand. He holds it up for me before putting it on the bedside table.
'Yeah?'
'Um…can I use your card again? To buy food? I need to go home to pick up my geography books for tomorrow, and Dad can't pick me up until eight. So, I need to buy something to eat.'
'Of course you can. Take whatever you need. I think there's also cash in the bedroom, in my bedside drawer. Use that.'
Luckily my boys are independent and responsible. I would trust Richard with anything of mine, and it may be that I will have to load much more onto his shoulders soon.

Richard looks at me, his young face serious, but I can also tell that he is anxious to leave. 'Are you sure you're going to be all right Mum, I mean if I go now? Do you want me to bring you anything tomorrow?'

Bless him. 'Honestly, I'm fine. I'm not going anywhere so there's nothing much I need anyway.' I roll my eyes upwards, referring to the various contraptions holding me down in bed, immobilised. 'You'd better run along, it's late. See you tomorrow. Kiss.'

A peck on the cheek and Richard is gone. I feel bad about not having been completely honest about my prognosis and I think back to my conversation with the doctors earlier. The medical team had come to see me early on, to let me know that they would need to operate. Doctor Kumar had explained the risks of the surgery. There was a distinct possibility that I would never walk again, that I would be confined to a wheelchair.

When he had finished, he asked me if I had any questions. I told him exactly what I thought – that if the operation failed and I could never walk again, then I would prefer to die during the operation. My words certainly had an impact on the medical team. Everyone had stared at me with horrified looks on their faces, frozen, not knowing what to say. Doctor Kumar seemed to look at me with disdain. I valued him as a doctor and a person, and I had felt deeply ashamed. What was wrong with me? Anybody else in my position would be hanging onto the smallest hope, not praying for a fast death.

This was the only reason why I had told Richard a sugared

version of my prospects for the future. I was scared that I might reveal to my son how badly I wanted to die, and risk him reacting in the same way as the doctors had this morning. I would not want to see that expression of horror and disgust on my son's face too.

3rd March 2005

The night before the operation I have a vision. It is dark, and the woman in the bed next to me is groaning constantly. Despite the doctors approving heavier pain medication, I cannot fall asleep. Now that the ward's daytime bustle has died down, the incessant symphony of the night time hospital – heart and blood pressure monitors, sighs, moans, bodily noises – is driving me mad. Ever since Doctor Kumar's visit, my brain has been working overtime. Frightened, desperate thoughts flying feverishly back and forth. These thoughts are wearing me out and I long for release, but there is nothing I can do. I am trapped in my own body.

I lose track of time and finally, thankfully, the painkillers begin to take the edge off. I don't like the haze the medication sends my way, but at night it doesn't matter so much. Perhaps now I can drift off.

I am not sure if I have fallen asleep for a short while, or just got lost in thought, but I come to, hearing a strange noise, a humming, or maybe ....chanting? It sounds so beautiful that I strain my ears to hear more. Has somebody left a radio on somewhere? After a while of listening intently, I give up. Maybe I dreamt it. I am about to close my eyes when I see a sudden flash of orange colour from the corner of my eye. What on earth was that? I hear whispering, like several people were talking at the same time. I hold my breath, moving my eyeballs from side to side, up and down, trying to see, but I can make out nothing in the darkness. 'Nurse?' No one answers. I lie there, alert now. The woman next to me says something in her sleep, then begins to snore very softly. The machines beep and tick.

Then, slowly, the room begins to spin around. Or perhaps my bed is spinning. Leisurely at first, it feels like lying on a lilo at a swimming pool on a warm summer's day. It's as if I were drifting gently in the softest of breezes. A beautiful singing begins to drift in from all around me. It sounds like it is coming from outside and inside of me at the same time – a chorus of male voices, a deep, lilting incantation. The language is foreign to me, but it doesn't seem to matter because I know the voices are singing about peace.

My bed continues to spin, or so it seems. Above me I see another streak of orange. It swoops past, making the hairs on my head move in its wake, and the singing increases in rhythm, rising up through my whole being, soothing. I smile and feel like joining the choir, but my voice will not work. I let go, and my soul joins in instead, a feeling of absolute calm coming over me. Another orange shape moves through the air, and this time it stays, drawing a beautiful spiral of gold above my head in anti-clockwise swirls. My bed spins faster and faster, like I was being sucked upwards into its centre. The orange colour begins to take shape. It spreads and morphs into separate splashes of colour above me which in turn begin to spread and shift and move, until human forms start to emerge from them. I stare, fascinated at the sight, my eyes open, not daring to blink in case these magical figures go away. I want them to stay. Have I died or is this real?

I see faces of men emerge, dressed in orange robes, heads shaved and bowed, chanting to the rhythm of a deep drum, walking slowly in step with its beat. My bed slows down and, as the spinning comes to a halt and I float in space, the men loom over me, singing and telling a story of hope, telling me that everything has a meaning, a place, a way. That is why they are here, to remind me of the road I have to take, the one that I have wandered away from.

In my head a word forms. T... A... O... Tao. The Way. Although I have never heard this word before, I know with certainty that these holy men are Taoists monks.

Then the spinning starts again, and quickly, faster and faster. The room, my bed, the entire universe is turning in lightning circles and the monks begin to blur and turn into darkness. With sadness I watch as the vision quivers and breaks up. Now I am falling into another spiral, a black hole that has opened up all around me. I am unable to resist its pull. As the murk swallows me into unconsciousness, I try to take the vision and the monks' song with me, but to my despair they seem to be slipping from my grasp, disappearing from my mind. What can I do? I want to remember... The last thought that enters my mind before I pass out is a certainty that, no matter what happens, I have to see these monks again. I have to remember their message. I believe somehow they will help me to recover, to walk again. I am sure that somehow the monks are significant. If I get another chance at life, if I have survived this far, then I must have a further purpose on this earth.

Surgery

I underwent surgery on the Tuesday. I told Richard of the possible consequences. He cried. I shouldn't have said anything. I remember the prepping, being taken down, being given the general anaesthetic...

The operation took over five hours.

A human neck has seven bones, C1 - C7. Doctor Kumar made an incision in the front of my neck to gain access. He fused C5 – C7 with titanium plates. He needed extra bone which he took from my right hip. To this day I have numbness in my right side and the fingers on my right hand are unable to grip well.

I came around. I didn't die on the table, as you'll have gathered. As I remembered where I was and what had just occurred, I was petrified. What if I was now completely paralysed? Dear reader, you may remember some big moments in your own life. Right there I had one of my biggest. I wiggled my big toe.

Ever since I had been scooped from the bottom of the stairs that night, I had worn a halo-type neck brace. I was to wear a neck brace for another six months. The marks remained on my skin long afterwards. The magician who is Doctor Kumar told me that the operation had been successful. It would, however, be a long road to recovery although I would get plenty of help. It would be mainly down to me and my determination.

I started flat on my back, motionless. Then, day by day, inch by inch, the staff inclined the top half of my bed. Eventually I started to see the room, see my fellow patients, got to know them a little. I started to move my legs, just because I could. Even this was hard work, but it gave me a huge sense of positivity, and of hope. 'Wow!' 'Amazing!' my fellow patients would cry. In return I tried to be as encouraging as I could. I learnt that, when you are at your lowest, the slightest ray of sunshine can help. 'Hey, sexy toenails!' went the porter, more than once. What a lift it gave me. I'd had a pedicure a few days earlier.

I even welcomed in my 'ants'. They were in my imagination of course, not in this spotless, hygienic hospital. My ants crawled all over my neck, my back. I knew that they were a sign of healing.

I treasured visiting time, seeing Richard and also my friends. All of this helped when I most needed it. Ten of the Crapaud Hash House Harriers came in to see me, causing havoc as they do everywhere. They made me laugh. I ask you, dear reader, if you know someone who is in a bad place, just say hello, touch base. It will mean more than you can know.

And, curiously, I had visits from Simon, the bloke who had walked away into the night when I fell down the stairs. He only visited outside normal visiting hours, almost like he didn't want to be seen. Although he voiced his concern about me, it seemed as if he was more concerned to absolve himself for his inaction that night. Maybe he thought I'd take some sort of action against him, as if I didn't have bigger things to worry about. It's all the same now anyway, he's no longer with us.

Eventually I was able to clamber out of bed, with help. I had a bed by a window so I didn't have to scramble too far to grip the cill and try to bend my legs. With support, I could look out of the window, see the sea. Difficult though this was, it was a signal that the hospital could do little more for me. It was suggested to me that I could leave when I wished, and of course full home support would be available. I didn't feel capable, no matter what help was available, but at the same time, I was realistic. I was taking up a bed which someone else might need.

So, a date was set and arrangements made. A few weeks after the operation, with Rachel as my carer, I was wheeled out into her car.

Challenges

'OK, I'm ready,' I said to Rachel.

She regarded me searchingly for a few seconds, the familiar, fun twinkle in her eye. 'Forget them next door. Your recovery is what's important now. They'll just have to deal with it. Who knows, you might need to build a ramp now!' Rachel walked towards me and squatted down, positioning herself below me at the bottom of the steps.

'What on earth are you doing?' I asked her. I could not look down to see but I saw a tuft of dark hair and heard her shoes crunching on the gravel. Then I felt her strong hands grabbing my ankles firmly. She pushed on them, upwards and in and, painstakingly, she helped me raise them up to the next step. She then walked up the stairs and squatted behind me, and then I felt two firm hands under my armpits again.

'OK?' she asked.

'Yes,' I replied, 'What are we doing?'

'Getting your bum onto the next step.'

'Ah.'

'Now. I'll count to three, and then all you need to do is try to push up with your legs and I'll help you up one step at a time.'

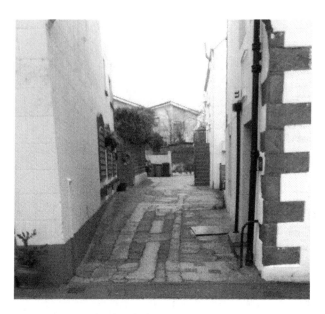

The dreaded steps, on the right

Concentrating my mind on the task ahead, I let Rachel count to three and pushed with all my might. Even though everything hurt as I strained my body upwards and back, Rachel's idea was working. We were in motion and I managed to get onto the next level.

'Good,' Rachel panted, 'now let's repeat.' With a big effort we made it to the top step. 'Now, into the house, all in one go,' Rachel instructed. We made headway slowly, my chest and underarms soaked with the effort and my breath was coming in short, raspy gasps. She was right behind me, stepping backwards, supporting my body with hers. 'Ouch, door,' she muttered as we crossed the threshold. She must have hit her elbow on the door frame, but I was too breathless to ask her if she was all right. The pain in my arms was now great. 'Only a bit to go now,' Rachel said. We approached the inside of the house. Despite the pain and exhaustion, the smell of my own home hit my nostrils and I breathed it in with pleasure. I had never realised that my house had a familiar smell until now. I had been in the sterile hospital environment for so long. It was heavenly.

We progressed through the lounge, Rachel clearly determined to get me into my chair. I could feel my heart pounding and I was sweating like a pig. For a moment I wondered if it was possible to have a heart attack from physical effort. I closed my eyes and willed myself on. One step, move backwards, pause. Another step, another. Inch by inch we made it through the lounge doorway, but then I thought that my lungs might burst.

'Wait, wait, got to rest...' We ground to a halt and I felt Rachel's body heat, her heavy breathing on my neck, her arms around my chest. A good job that she was this strong and fit. We had rowed together for years and our combined upper-body strength was now being used in a way never intended.
'OK, let's carry on, I told her.

We started again, inching on, and eventually made it to the chair. This was a special, straight-back padded chair that had been delivered especially for me by Family Nursing and Home Care. I was to see a lot of it. Carefully we began to turn around, like a clumsy couple learning to waltz for the first time. Soon I was positioned with my back to the chair, feeling the footrest against my ankle. Rachel moved me to one side to let me position myself as best I could. I instinctively put my arms out, but then realised they were useless for supporting my weight. Rachel grunted and lowered me down as slowly as she could. My sweating had reached epic proportions by now but I landed in the chair and finally able to breathe, took in a huge breath of air and let it out. I was properly, definitely home.

Home again

I managed. Goodness knows how. Everything was a major effort. I simply would have failed without the nurses from Family Nursing and Home Care, a Jersey-based charity. They came every day to help me with mobility exercises, checking me over, washing and bathing, doing my shopping, a hundred things that all of us take for granted when we're well. I also had Richard who couldn't have been more caring at an age where he shouldn't have been expected to.

Poor Richard, I thought. He was fed up with looking after me, day after day. I was fed up too. I felt guilty, but, even so, thought about my new idea again. My arms couldn't lift a book or magazine high enough. My hands weren't strong enough to hold a book for long. I couldn't bend my neck to look down. If only I had a music stand that would make life a lot easier.

He came back into the room carrying two cups of tea. 'Right. Do you need me to do anything else before I go upstairs? Like, not a music stand...' He put my tea cup, with a straw sticking out of it, on a coaster on my little table next to my chair.
'Thank you for everything Richard. You are wonderful.' He

nodded curtly, but I thought I could see the hint of a smile on his lips as he turned and left the room.

Make dinner, wash clothes, do the dishes, close the curtains, turn off the telly, new loo roll, bring me my medicine, turn off the light, could you just…, would you please… My youngest, I thought, must be at the end of his tether. All the mundane things I used to do without even thinking. It really was unfair on Richard and I felt very guilty. I'd ask Maggie or Rachel about the music stand.

> *Richard says, 'That was a very difficult year or so for both of us. I have an abiding image of those days – Mum's upright, turquoise chair. She would sit in it all day long. Even when she wasn't in it, the chair would sit there as some awful beacon, a symbol of us both being trapped, imprisoned.*
>
> *'I'd get up in the mornings. Mum's hands were so bad that she could do very little for herself. I'd make her a cup of tea. Then I'd chop vegetables, open tins, make sure everything was as easy as possible for her. In the evening I'd go shopping, make sure we had enough stuff in the house. I was 17, learning on the hoof, making it up as I went along.'*

André, my eldest, was at university so by unfair default, my youngest was left to look after his mother. Thank goodness he was so competent as well as kind. He cooked and cleaned without having to be asked. He even massaged my arms every day, to relax them, ease the pain. Richard will recall giving me Chinese Burns. You may remember giving or receiving such minor torture in your own school days. I found that, together with the massage, it helped the pain enormously. Poor Richard though, it really was too much for a 17-year old.

André says 'I was in my first year at Bournemouth when I heard about Mum's accident. I immediately went to see my tutor to arrange to go home. He refused, point blank. He even implied that I was lying in order to get time off. There was not a shred of support or sympathy from the university. This shocked me and affected my attitude towards the institution for the rest of my time there.

'I was also pretty broke. I spoke to Dad and Richard. The consensus was that no purpose would be served by me returning home immediately. Mum was in the best possible place. I'd return home during the next university break.

'So I never saw Mum in hospital. When I came home I saw that Richard had effectively become her carer. I felt excluded, alien and guilt-ridden. It was my first major life crisis.'

Together with the wonderful nurses at Family Nursing and Home Care, Richard was ensuring that I was slowly getting my life back. Without everybody's help I would probably have had to stay in hospital. Rachel came around frequently to keep me company. Maggie was a professional carer and she would come and give me massages as well as company.

Maggie would say 'aren't you doing well', or 'you are so positive.' My friends were a constant comfort and source of encouragement.

Another man who appeared like an angel was Peter Tregloan. Those interested in elite powerlifting and Strongman events will recognise the name. Peter is a big, big man and he was extraordinarily successful as a powerlifter. He was World Super Heavyweight Champion no fewer than nine times, and still holds records in Masters categories. He represented Great Britain, and indeed Jersey, many times in Strongman competition. Yet this big man has the gift of healing and has helped many elite lifters and other sportsmen and women. The Cranio Sacral Therapy that he did with me in those dark days helped enormously. Peter now lives in his native Cornwall but still visits Jersey occasionally. I visited him recently for another session and to thank him for his support.

I'd spend those days, and bleak days they were, pretty much immobile in my upright chair. There was a window to look out of, but nothing to see – rooftops, clouds – though the sea front was only a minute or two away. But one day, suddenly there were mountains. Yes, mountains outside my window. Not clouds shaped like mountains. They were actual mountains, brown with patches of green glinting in the sunlight, reaching to the sky. Inviting, tempting. I gazed at them, entranced, for several minutes. Then they were gone. Much as I willed them to, the mountains never came back, as with the Taoist monks. But, each in their own way, they turned out to be more prophetic than I could ever have known.

'Mum?' I turned towards the door. Richard was in the lounge doorway, proffering a blue box in my direction. 'I'm having biscuits with my tea. Want one?'

'Good idea, thank you. Ooh, Oreos. Just one please.' He placed an Oreo on a napkin next to my teacup. 'Richard, thank you for looking after me so well. I know it must be hard. It won't go on forever. As soon as I can I'll be doing things for myself. It's driving me mad as well.'

'No worries.' He paused for a moment as if about to say something. Then he changed his mind and left the room again, muttering something that sounded like 'homework'.

I tested my tea again. It had cooled down so I raised it carefully to my lips with both hands. It was lovely – warm and sweet. As I lowered it back down, a little crack appeared in the clouds and the sun came out for a few fleeting seconds. It filled the room and made the lounge look brighter and happier. Then it disappeared again. Sunlight changes everything. I wished that I could have more of it.

> *Richard says, 'I began to wonder when it would all end. The thing with the Chinese Burns I used to give Mum. It gave her some relief in an odd way. This, the constant caring, became my life and I grew to resent it. After a while I used to get agitated, annoyed, though I knew I shouldn't. It was a year of sadness, of regret, of fear for the future. When Mum started to improve with therapy it was a great relief.*
>
> *'In later years I've begun to understand that I allocate a certain amount of patience to everyone. I have lots of patience with new people. My patience with Mum*

ran out long ago. She understands that, and knows I love
her despite this. We have a good, frank relationship and
we're both happy with that.'

Another helping hand

The phone rang and the nurse picked it up. 'Sandra's phone,
Linda speaking.' After a few seconds she handed the phone
to me. 'It's Olive, Frank's wife, from the Hash or
something?' Yes, Olive. I kind of knew her. I knew Frank
from my running days with the Hash House Harriers. Olive
was usually around arranging things, handing out
sandwiches, though I didn't know her all that well. Maybe
she was calling to ask for a bit of help at a forthcoming run.
I'd have to disappoint her.
'Hi Olive, how are you?'
'Hello dear. Glad you remember me. Your friend Rachel may
have warned you that I might ring. I just found out about
your accident. I must come and see you. Where do you
live?'

We arranged that she would call around the
following afternoon. I awaited her arrival, having given up
hope of finding anything to watch on the TV. I looked out of
the window, it was just as interesting as the TV. Grey clouds
again. I longed for sunshine.

Olive arrived on the dot of 3pm. Linda had gone. Olive
immediately made us both a cup of tea and had then pulled
up a chair close to mine. Opposite me, so I didn't need to
move my neck in the slightest. Her legs wide apart, her
strong thighs bulging inside her tracksuit bottoms. I had
never seen Olive in anything but sportswear.

We talked. I told Olive of my woes – the constant pain in my arms and neck, numbness in my legs. Above all, the interminable nights, lying down flat on my back, unable to change position, unable to sleep.

'Don't they give you pain medication?'

'Yes, but you've no idea of the side effects of that stuff. They are powerful, they do a good job with the pain, but, if I take them, I can do nothing else. I dare not even walk, I feel so drowsy. I need to walk properly again. Right now, that's my main goal in life. No, I've binned the painkillers.' I could have added that the pain reminded me of life before my accident. It was a strange motivation to concentrate on my recovery, on my new life. I needed to be free of all drugs in my body so I could feel the pain – if it was stronger or weaker – so I could feel if I was improving instead of just existing like a vegetable, on medication. I enjoyed feeling the 'ants' crawling through my body as I felt like I was healing.

'May I ask what exactly happened to you?' I was surprised that Rachel had not told her.

'In a nutshell, I broke my neck. Fell down the stairs.' I told her the story, glossing over the details.

'So you can walk a small distance, just not far? And your arms and hands work a little?'

'Yes, that's right.'

'But you are in a lot of pain.' I nodded.

'Rachel said you used to do rowing?'

'Yes, I loved rowing. It was my passion. I can show you some photographs. We won competitions and everything. That's all finished now of course.'

'Hmm,' Olive tilted her head at me. 'So, you enjoyed being on the water?'

My attempt at a brave smile didn't fool Olive. She smiled kindly, took my hand, patted it. I was embarrassed at my faux bravery being seen through so readily by a relative stranger. I tried again. 'So that's that. No rowing, but as soon as I'm moving again, I'll probably take up some form of activity. I've done yoga before, maybe that, when I'm stronger.'

Olive was nodding enthusiastically now. 'You're thinking along the same lines as me, I think. Now I know how I could help.' She proceeded to tell me her idea. It was brilliant. Why had I not thought of it myself? It was obvious. There were a few things to check, questions to ask, which I would do. I would then get back to Olive who would be my driver and companion for the day.

We chatted a little more, but I was now anxious to make some calls, to advance the plan. Fingers crossed, I could soon tell Richard that I would be out of his hair for a few afternoons here and there. I was excited.

In My Element

The machine made a smooth humming sound as I travelled up and away from the platform, swaying a couple of feet above ground. John called out, as he always did, 'All OK up there?'

'Yes, thank you,' I shouted back. Everything was more than OK, I thought happily as I gently swung from side to side in the aluminium harness chair. It was all fabulous. I was about to enjoy what had become my favourite pursuit of all time – the swimming pool.

This was about the sixth time that Olive had brought me to Les Quennevais Sports Centre, and their pool. Already I felt like an old hand, becoming accustomed to the crane, and to the swimming monitors who would help me in and out of the harness. The pool had become my new obsession. Every time Olive and I scheduled a visit, I would spend the whole week looking forward to it. Water was bliss.

There had been huge improvements in my mobility since I'd started these sessions. I doubt that physiotherapy alone could have achieved the results I was now enjoying. The muscle tone and the strength in my legs had increased since I started. I had also discovered that being in water greatly alleviated the excruciating cramps and stabbing pains which still persisted in my arms and neck since the operation. I still resisted the heavy-duty pain meds. The pool was now the one place where my physical discomfort became manageable, and for minutes at a time I was pain-free.

My toes hit the water. I'd been so deep in thought I'd quite forgotten where I was. I took in the sensations as the chair swayed lower and my ankles and calves were immersed in the tepid water. Then my knees and thighs. Finally, my toes touched the bottom of the pool. Then the aluminium chair to which I was strapped wobbled. I waited for it to gently settle onto all four of its supporting legs before I began to undo the supporting harness.

The staff at the pool were fantastic. They could not have been more helpful. They were ever watchful, making sure that I was not in trouble. As soon as I put my hand up, they would help me back out of the pool. Then Olive, who did her Aqua Fit class while I waded, would help me back to the changing rooms and drive me back home. I was grateful to have so many incredibly helpful people around me. They all contributed to my recovery and would ensure that it was as quick as possible.

The side of the pool was only two easy steps away. I put my arms forward to support myself on the railing there. It was marvellous how everything felt so easy here. I was wearing a buoyancy belt and my body seemed almost weightless in the water. Compared to my heavy trudging on land, moving around in the pool was child's play. My legs could carry my body mass effortlessly.

The exercise I had prescribed myself consisted of walking from one end of the pool to the other. The first time I had tried, I had only made it to the other end and back before feeling totally exhausted. Then I had gradually added length, working on lifting my legs as high as possible, letting my arms feel the resistance of the water as I ploughed forward. Today I was aiming for a minimum of six lengths, adding a new element – punching the water ahead of me as I walked.

I remained at the side of the pool for a moment longer, just enjoying the sensations, feeling my feet on the tiles, listening to the murmur of a group of pensioner swimmers chatting by the poolside, the waves from the children's corner slapping against the filter openings. For a moment I shut my eyes. The atmosphere at the pool made me peaceful inside and I couldn't help smiling with contentment.

'Come on Sandra, time to get to work. You won't get there unless you put in the work.'

Fuengirola (Malaga)

Oh, I have slipped the surly bonds of earth,
And danced the skies on laughter-silvered wings
(John Gillespie Magee)

I have always loved travelling. When I was younger,
I yearned to escape the surly bonds of the grey north-west. I
watched travel programmes on the telly, devoured
magazines. The odd trip to Blackpool or Colwyn Bay was just
a tease, a taste of what might lie beyond my home territory.
When I eventually slipped those bonds, Jersey fitted the bill
perfectly. I immediately found freedom and was able to
begin to spread my wings.

Now, 11 months after my accident, Jersey had lost
its glamour and sheen. It was not poor Jersey's fault of
course. I was slow to complain – after all I had dodged both
death and an unthinkable lifetime of immobility. Jersey's
winters can be as bleak as anywhere in Britain, and my
mood was low in the early weeks of 2006. I was stuck at my
room at Maggie's, unable to drive, not able to walk far with
my stick. Something needed to change. Yes, I was far from
fully recovered but I was able to travel. With assistance,
certainly, as far as transport was concerned, but such
assistance is usually forthcoming, especially with forward
planning.

I felt I needed a bit of sunshine. My body
continually ached and I was sure the cold, damp winter was
doing nothing to help the matter. Why Spain? I'm really not

sure why I came to that decision. I know that my mind was still hazy from my meds and many of my actions at that time owed more to spontaneity rather than thought and planning. Spain, I knew, was sunny and well-known for being a winter retreat for Brits. Malaga is in the extreme south of Spain on the playground which is the Costa del Sol. My friend Jackie and me did some research and eventually decided to book ourselves on a yoga retreat there.

Off we went – au revoir Jersey, hola Spain! The Lemon Tree Farmhouse is a short distance from Malaga. We were picked up by the two sweet lesbian women who ran the retreat. A short drive maybe, but Pizarra was a different world from the busy coastal resort. Here were the mountains which I had seen from my window in First Tower! Rugged mountains, dusty plane trees with their hardy shrubbery and insect life. Green eucalyptus forests near lakes. High, clear blue skies. Having only seen coastal Andalucía before, this was a revelation.

A pleasant couple of weeks we spent at the Lemon Tree – doing yoga, being massaged, eating and drinking well, generally relaxing. Soaking up the sun, just what the doctor ordered. At the end of the two weeks Jackie decided to head back but...I wasn't ready to leave, just when I was starting to feel a little better, both physically and mentally. Jersey was still where I called home but I knew that my recovery would be best served here. I was falling in love with Spain. For the moment anyway I could afford to stay a little longer. Richard was perfectly independent now and didn't need me. André was still at university.

I took a short trip down the coast on the train to Fuengirola. No particular reason, but at this time I was often acting on impulse. I was never like that before the accident. Maybe my subconscious was now reminding me that we all have a finite number of years here on Earth, and no one can tell exactly how many we each have left. Yes, a clever actuary will calculate a life expectancy, but I had been damn close to upsetting those calculations at the age of 49. Now, a year later, I was starting off on Life #2 and my subconscious, my psyche, was urging me to make the most of it. Who knows when Life #2 might end.

Why Fuengirola I have no idea. These resorts on the Costa aren't everyone's cup of tea. Like many, it developed quickly from the 1960s onwards, with many high-rises, and no one can claim the town is beautiful. Yes, there is a little history, parks, the lovely old port. The long, golden beach, the promenade – the Paseo Maritimo Rey de España – are the focal points of the town, plus of course the dazzling sunshine which is basically endless in this part of the world.

After that short trip I went back to the Lemon Tree, but shortly afterwards decided to return to Fuengirola for a while. I decided to rent a flat. Looking back now, a 3-bed was too big really. I suppose I envisaged the boys and friends coming to visit. It was another indication, I guess, that I no longer saw Jersey as being my permanent home. The flat was at Los Boliches, one of Fuengirola's most famous beaches. I packed my stuff and left it at my new flat. I then decided that I really ought to return to Jersey, show my face at least. In fact, I travelled back more than once while I was living in Spain.

At this time I had sold the house at First Tower and was basically living off the proceeds. My base when in Jersey was still at Maggie's which I still rented. It was always good to come back to see the boys and my friends, but the Costa and the sunshine was calling and that's where I headed back.

As mentioned, the flat at Los Boliches, Fuengirola was lovely, but it really was too big. While leafing through the local paper I spotted an ad, one of many I suppose. Again, I seemed to be on some sort of pre-destined path and I just followed my instinct. The ad was for a flat share, and it was very close by. I loved the area and didn't want to move too far. The woman that had the flat was Georgina and I went to see it. Well, Georgina and I could have been twins. She also wasn't in the best of shape and when we met, both walking with sticks, it was a match made in heaven

We got on well, me and Georgina, but soon it was clear that her flat was too small for both of us, especially as Georgina was one of life's untidy people. So began the gypsy part of my life! Georgina said that she was thinking about buying a caravan. Off we went on our sticks to see the caravan – it was on a site two minutes from the beach. She bought it and moved in. After a short time she mentioned that the caravan next to hers was for sale. To cut a long story short, I bought the caravan and moved in next door to her, letting my previous flat go.

✈

The caravan was quite the affair, with all its trappings, probably not what you would normally expect at a camp site. The caravan itself was a battered, two-berth 90s Autosleeper. It was permanently parked on the right-hand side of my allocated 12 x 7 metre plot. Attached to, and covering the side where the main cabin door opened onto the plot was a large rectangular tent the width and height of a reasonably large and airy room. Made of hardy, rubber-coated canvas, it was waterproof and kept the wind out efficiently. Strapped tightly onto the caravan's roof and sides it was held in shape by thick aluminium poles and several sturdy metal wires. It took over about a third of the plot, and it served as my front room.

The bedroom was inside the caravan itself. It was set up with all the mod-cons – air conditioning both in the caravan and also in the tent. A big TV with satellite connection for Sky in the tent. A DVD player, sound system, comfy sofa, coffee table and a desk for my laptop. My neighbour even had WiFi and let me have the password in return for a small monthly donation.

When I had been negotiating the purchase of this wonder in modern camping, I had initially been concerned about thieves getting into such a flimsy structure, but the lady who had sold it had assured me that as long as I locked the smaller valuables in the caravan, and kept my passport on me, then the larger items would be completely safe. The camp site security and the tall fence surrounding the site made it impossible for bulky items to be carried away. Also, many of those living on the site had been there for many years. Strangers were quickly noticed. As long as you made yourself known to your neighbours, they would look out for you. She had convinced me.

Next to me lived a couple, Bryan and Sheila. On a camp site you soon get to know your neighbours and I'm happy to say that I'm still in touch with them today. It turned out that Bryan was a faith healer. Ever since my accident I had been in chronic pain, to a greater or lesser degree. I was open to anything that would ease the pain, make my life a little more comfortable. Medicinal painkillers did, of course, have a part to play, especially in the early part of my recovery. Though I'm no medic, I knew that relying on painkillers were no long-term solution if I was to lead any sort of 'normal' life. They made me drowsy and unable to function properly. Also, I was well aware that my body would soon become normalised to ordinary painkillers and I would need stronger and stronger stuff. I didn't wish to go down that road, especially remembering my father was on 21 different opioids when he died.

Fortunately, I have (or was acquiring) a very open mind. And various therapies had indeed brought about improvements. Faith healing was something I was keen to try. And I struck lucky with Bryan. He came over on a daily basis and did light massage. They were both a great comfort to me, and assisted me generally at that time. Funnily it turns out that I might have a touch of magic hands myself – they seemed to work on my son Richard when he had a bad knee. Maybe I inherited a little of this healing, and second sight, from my mother's Irish roots. In old Ireland it was accepted without question that some people had the 'Gift' or the 'Sight'. (The Irish weren't so zealous about eliminating witches during the 16th and 17th centuries as in other places. Most unexplained happenings were attributed instead to the faeries!)

A trip to the masseur

At 9.30 this morning I had hiked all the way into town, planning to go to the bank, the supermarket, the Telecom shop to make some calls, and then for my bi-weekly massage session with Jens, my hulking Dutch masseur with the strongest hands on earth, who I had found through my yoga contacts. He had done some great work on my shoulders and arms up until now.

The bank had been full of people with only one clerk at the window and a queue of people all breathing down each other's necks. By the time I had reached the cashier and withdrawn some money it was 11.30 and I was seriously fed up and tired. I still needed to go to the supermarket before seeing the masseur, but the telephone calls would have to wait for another day.

'Excuse me, I'm next!' The two ladies pushing in front of me at the cheese counter turned around and eyed me up sullenly, but seeing my posture, stood back. What was it this morning? People were trampling all over me. Only when I had got angry and shouldered in, waving my little numbered ticket and demanding to be served had they reluctantly given way. Why do they bother with numbers in the first place if no one uses them? The petulant girl on the counter had served me as slowly and silently as she could, as if I had insulted her personally with my strange foreign ways.

Eventually, by now muttering to myself, I got my quarter of cheese, rushed to pay at the till, and set off towards the clinic. It was only when I got there, sweaty and stressed, that I realised that I had forgotten to buy bread. Oh well, there was nothing I could do about it right now. 'There's a bakery down the road,' the receptionist explained sympathetically from behind the desk as I undressed and recounted my woes to her.

'That's no good for me. It will be closed by the time I finish here.'

'True,' she agreed, showing me into the treatment room. He'll be with you in a moment. Just take off your clothes and lie down under this towel.'

Never mind, I consoled myself, struggling with my bra. I'll get some from the camp site shop later. The horrible, tough, chewy bread from the camp shop was not the best, but needs must I suppose.

Still stressed, I had laid down on the massage table for my treatment, and things then went from bad to worse. Jens, the masseur I liked was not in and the man who came to give me my treatment just didn't hit the mark. It had turned out to be the most painful session that I had ever experienced. It was not his fault, but for some reason all my nerve endings seemed to be giving me anxiety.

In fact, when I thought about it, the 'good' sensations in the back of my neck (like ants walking up and down my spine) which I had learnt to welcome and associate with healing, had not been present for a few days now. I had desperately wanted some relief, but somehow the whole session had felt tortuous. Eventually, after enduring it for about half an hour, I decided to cut my losses. 'I just can't get comfortable today. Sorry, it's not your fault. Today just isn't a good day.'

I could tell the masseur felt disappointed but he agreed, very kindly, to charge me for only half a session. 'I'll call you a taxi,' he said, after putting the money in a little box in the reception drawer and sliding it closed. The receptionist had gone for lunch.

'No thank you, I'll walk. Got to get my exercise somehow.'

Happily, the bakery was still open when I walked past and I was able to get a loaf of soft bread to take home with me. I was pleased that at least something had worked out.

About half-way back to the camp site, I began to realise I ought to have accepted the offer of a taxi home. I was struggling. I usually had my massage session in the evening, and the air was considerably cooler then. Now, with the sun at its zenith and the cool morning air long gone, a scorching heat had taken its place.

Fifteen minutes later I struggled onto my makeshift porch at the camp site – six wooden slats laid out onto the bare earth with a green tarpaulin strung overhead for shade. I felt very faint. This was not just an ordinary dizzy spell and I began to sway. I dropped the supermarket bag on the floor – there was a cracking sound as it hit the wooden deck. There go the eggs, I thought fuzzily as I reached for the nearest plastic chair. I more or less fell into the chair, sideways, painfully, the plastic legs bending and scratching against the floor. I tried to get the blood flowing back into my head by putting it as far between my knees as my spine would allow, which was not far at all. Hunched over, I sat there for a while. My shoulders and arms were throbbing, and I could feel the metal plate under the skin in my upper spine pressing and constricting my movement. For a minute I thought that I might throw up.

Then I remembered to try and breathe into the areas of pain, like the Lemon Tree yoga teacher had taught me. I tried to sit more comfortably and began to take slow breaths, following the air through my nose and into my lungs, and out again through my nose, slowly, deliberately. Almost straight away the nausea began to subside. The dizziness had completely passed now. I straightened up, stretched my back, blowing out a final and deliberate puff of breath. 'Right, let's get you sorted.' Standing up carefully I tested my legs. When I found them working, I picked up the shopping bag from the floor and checked for broken eggs. Only one. I took the grocery bag over to the back of my porch, to the rather bizarre, but very useful, feature of my temporary home – a fully fitted kitchen, installed outside the tent and as an extension to my 'porch'. It was great. Despite looking like Ikea had driven by here and accidentally dumped a show kitchen on the caravan grounds and then sped off, the kitchen was fully functional with an oven, running tap water and a fridge. It was connected to the camp site's electricity, running water and drainage hook-ups, found on each plot, and the porch's tarpaulin roof shielded it from the rain (which of course was rare).

I put the food away in the cupboards and the fridge, cleaning the traces of the broken egg away. Satisfied, I turned around and entered my front room through the flap that served as a door and walked across to the caravan door, slinging my sunglasses on the writing desk on the way past. Then I carefully climbed up the treacherously narrow front steps of the Autosleeper.

Turning the key in the lock, I knew what to expect when I opened the door. Inside, the air was so hot that the tiny space felt more like an oven than somewhere humans might live. Nevertheless, I clambered in and, finding the remote for the air conditioning unit, switched it on high, leaving the door wide open. To Hell with the environment, it would survive five minutes until I was properly cooled down.

Slowly and gingerly, I peeled off my damp t-shirt. Every move was laborious and unpleasant after this morning's rough massage, but eventually the sweaty item went into the laundry bag. Then, as an afterthought, because I could not get cool quickly enough, so did the rest of my clothing. It was too hot to put a robe on, and so I shut the caravan door and grabbed an ice-cold bottle of water from the fridge. Then I finally allowed myself onto the window seat.

Sitting down felt wonderful. I moved around until I found a comfortable position against the pillows I had laid on the back rest so that I could sit here comfortably straight. I allowed myself to relax and enjoy, closing my eyes and sighing contentedly. After a while I opened my eyes and rubbed them. My skin felt dusty and I knew that I should really take a shower before the sweat dried, but I just wanted to sit here for a moment more in the slowly cooling air. Thanks to the fitted kitchen outside, the shower inside the Autosleeper was rendered useless, and trekking all the way to the camp site shower right now was about as appealing as trekking through the Gobi Desert. Maybe I should ask the camp site manager if I could sort out another water connection, I pondered idly. The aircon was kicking in now, blowing cool air that tickled my arm.

Finally, blissfully, I fell asleep.

A visit from Rachel

It was great to see my old running and rowing partner when she came down for a visit. But let Rachel tell the story in her own words.

> Rachel says, 'I went to Fuengirola for Sandra's 50th birthday, for a long weekend. It was a very wet and stormy weekend too - it didn't stop raining the whole time. Sandra was living on a caravan park at the time. She had a lovely little van decorated out in her very own style. We visited her friend Georgina who was in hospital. Fencing and awnings were blown down in the caravan park during the storms and we (Sandra said it was just me) helped put those back. We went out for dinner with some friends, Bryan & Sheila. I bought her a silver links charm bracelet for her birthday, she then told me she couldn't bear anything on her wrists! Sandra drove me back to the airport and that was when the sun started to shine!'

The boys come to stay

I was delighted when Richard, having just finished university, came down to Malaga. It was the first of many visits to wherever I happened to be. He fitted right in to the beach culture and the area generally. He rented a house in Puerto Banus. Naturally he soon got involved with the local cycling club, and taught himself Spanish. He also took a massage course in Fuengirola. It was never to be a long term move and Richard returned to Jersey.

André also came to stay in the caravan after university, and he stayed for a while when I returned to Jersey. I think it was a bit boring for him – not too many young people, and he needed to learn the language to work there.

Both André and Richard were to visit me regularly in the years to come, wherever I happened to be. I'm blessed to have these boys.

I might have given the impression that I had forgotten all about Jersey. Far from it. During my two years in Malaga I would often hop back to visit. Jersey was still my domicile of choice (as they say in tax speak) and I still had lots of friends back home.

It was during one of these trips that I began to feel restless again. As good as Malaga had been to me there was no reason for me to make my relationship with it a permanent one. I was still in the early stages of my Life#2 as I was beginning to see it. I was young, so much to see and do. I still needed the sunshine though, and access to sea bathing and a choice of local and affordable therapies. I discussed the matter with Maggie and she was happy to throw around possibilities with me. I had visited Mallorca once or twice and something about it appealed to me. Years before my accident, a clairvoyant had said that I'd live in Mallora in the future. Whether that was in the back of my mind or not I couldn't say.

'Well, go to Mallorca then,' said Maggie.

'I think I might. I'd like to drive there.' I still owned my old faithful blue Ford Escort Cabriolet.

'Drive? Why? Anyway you can't, you're not strong enough. Your hands, your shoulders...'

'No, but you can.'

'What!'

And so it was that we made our preparations. I still had my caravan and belongings in Fuengirola, and I was still renting my room at Maggie's. Here I was, heading off somewhere else, this time with my good friend.

The great day came. We'd packed everything we needed. We looked at it, we then looked at the car. It would never all fit. We tried anyway, packing in stuff as best we could. Still plenty to go, Maggie climbed into the passenger seat. I continued to cram stuff in on top of her. Somehow we managed and off we set.

We drove down through France. In the end I ended up doing much of the driving as it was mainly motorway and easy driving. It was OK, the French main roads are easy to drive on. We stayed over at a chateau near Bordeaux and continued on the next day, reaching Barcelona in the early evening. From there we would catch the ferry to Mallorca but we would stay in Barcelona overnight. Happily, disabled badge holders appeared to be well catered for and, a little way from our chosen hotel, was a disabled bay. We parked and slept the sleep of the righteous.

Next day the car was gone! In its place were, apparently, instructions as to how to proceed. In Spanish. My familiarity with the language was basic and of no use in this situation. Panicking was no use so we accosted an innocent passer-by who translated for us and pointed out the way to the car pound. It was there that we learnt the difference between 'public disabled' and 'private disabled'. Despite our protests of innocence, we were fined 90 euros, which I considered a reasonable result. Best not to confront the Spanish cops, they will always win. It was fine.

Escaping from mainland Spain we arrived in Mallorca later that day. I was to live there, on and off, for the next four years.

Mallorca

I walk in the sunshine
You live in the night
You're not where I'm going
The future is bright
I'll live in the sunshine
I've chosen the light
(Adeline Foster)

I soon settled down. I am an adaptable animal, or at least I am proving to be in Life#2. I rented a cheap flat, so I now laid claim to:

Maggie's flat in Jersey
My caravan in Fuengirola, Malaga
My small flat in Puerto Portals, the glamour hotspot of Mallorca, on the coast between the capital Palma and Magaluf.

This may make me sound as if I'm Lady Rockefeller or the Queen of Sheba, but really I lived quite frugally. I don't drink or smoke, not in my new life anyway. Others can do as they wish but my damaged body needs all the help it can get. Booze and fags don't come into that category. Neither do I party or frequent expensive restaurants – unless someone else is paying of course. (Joke, I'm not that bad.)

Maggie didn't stay long in Mallorca. That was never the plan in any case. Her life was in Jersey. There was a gym just across the road from my flat, perfect. I would go across there and do some light exercise, use the pool at the flat, which I used to enjoy.

This is a good opportunity to explain about my spinning CDs. When I was recovering from my accident in Jersey I was living in Maggie's flat, often tired with nothing to do. I've always enjoyed music, especially that of my teens and early 20s years. I decided to make up music compilation CDs. This was way before I ever thought of teaching spinning classes. It wasn't that, but I somehow knew that they would become useful in future years.

So, over time, I made over 30 CDs. I still have them and use them to this day. To give you an idea, here of some of the artistes that you can expect if you listen to them.

Yazz (The Only Way is Up) of course, Chris Rea, Bryan Adams, Lighthouse Family, Otis Redding Kool & the Gang, Freda Payne, Smokey Robinson & the Miracles, Commodores, Michael Jackson, Dolly Parton, Craig David, Geri Halliwell, Gloria Gaynor, Shania Twain, Rod Stewart, Sade, Anastacia, Simon & Garfunkel, Eternal, Shakin' Stevens, Tom Jones, U2, Martha Reeves, Free, Wet Wet Wet, Phil Collins, Various Motown classics, Status Quo, and many more.

So anyway, I had my CDs with me in Mallorca. Acting (as ever in Life#2) on impulse I enquired of the owner if I might possibly teach a spinning class. She was dubious but I was doing it for free, so I was allocated the room on Saturday mornings. At my first class there were four or five old people. Then a few younger ones started to come. After a month the class was full – they were loving it. I'm continually told how much people love the music. At this stage it was all still unpaid, though eventually I asked, and got, a few euros. It was never about the money; I was doing it for myself. I loved it, and still enjoy leading spinning classes to this day as it's a great form of exercise.

✈

Returning to those hard days in Jersey after my accident, I had many strange thoughts. It was as if my brain had been nudged into a different gear. I thought about things that would never have crossed my mind beforehand. This sixth sense, or intuition, has become almost natural to me now. One of these passing thoughts was that I should start a Ladies' Club, somewhere for women to meet socially. Don't ask me why. After I'd decided on Mallorca (with Maggie's help) I researched the subject of women's clubs there. I even, with André's help, set up a website.

Sure enough, I got to know lots of lovely people in Mallorca. The time was right. I set up Mallorca Ladies Club, and, for a while, it became my life. It was a once-a-month thing, a social gathering for 'ladies who lunch'. I didn't make money from it, that was never my intention. I did make lifelong friends. And I also became well known down there, appearing in glossy magazines and such. As before, I made several trips to and from Jersey over those three years, a good job I enjoy flying, and having assistance makes it easier.

It was through the Ladies Club that I found a new place to live. One of the many women I met there happened to mention that she had an apartment to let – would I like to see it? I was happy enough where I was but popped along for a look anyway. It was down nearer the port of Portals and It was huge, three bedrooms, and cheap too! Well I had to take it. It was great for a time. I was able to have family and friends visit, it was in the lively port area. I was even able to start hosting my Ladies Club there. But I had been wrong to mix my personal life with the Ladies Club. All of a sudden it didn't feel like my home any more. Suddenly the rent demanded went through the roof. I moved on.

Moved on, but not far. Portals village is typical Spanish and I found a lovely, quiet one-bedroom place there, with even a little garden. It was here that I tried something a little different, a Singles Club – Mallorca Solos. We decided to invite single men as well. It was fun. We'd meet at various bars to drink, eat, chat but without any pressure to pair off, anything like that. (Though what happened afterwards I wouldn't know.)

Not name dropping or anything, but one of our regular meeting places was a bar often frequented by Peter Stringfellow, who'd be there with his wife perhaps, or at least a woman, happily passing the time of day. Also Pauline Quirke, of *Birds of a Feather* fame, who has lent her name to an academy for the performing arts in the town.

There were visits to the capital, Palma, which was 30 minutes away by bus, always with an eye out for a good massage therapist there. One such was Bendy Wendy, also an exponent and teacher of yoga as you might have guessed.

Of personal relationships in Mallorca there may have been one or two. There springs to mind Erik the Swedish priest. We became friends and I'd meet him, and sometimes accompany him to weddings on the island. He's happily married these days, living back in Sweden, and we're still occasionally in touch.

Florida – Carrots and Spinning

As I've mentioned, each of these longer sojourns to Spain and its islands were frequently punctuated by trips, either back to Jersey or further afield. In 2010 I took a trip to Florida. One of the many people I met via the Ladies Club was Beverley Pugh. We got chatting (if there was an Olympics for chatting then I'd qualify automatically). One of our common interests was in alternative therapies. I was intrigued when Beverley described her raw food regime and the benefits it brought. Renewed energy, clearer skin, better digestion, better health generally. Everyone is aware that eating more natural whole foods and less processed food is a good idea generally. An exclusive raw food diet would simply be an extension of this. I gave it a go for a while and indeed I felt better in myself.

I read up a little bit on the subject hoping maybe to find something akin to the yoga retreat which I'd found so beneficial in Malaga. Yes of course there were any number of health resorts, wellness retreats and suchlike, all promising to transform your life, for a price. None of these places hopes or expects to attract those of limited means. I was fortunate in that I was even able to consider such an indulgence. I'm far from rich but I was willing to push the boat out as far as my health and well-being was concerned.

I scanned, skimmed, read. I kept coming back to one website in particular. The Hippocrates Health Institute in West Palm Beach, Florida promised to cure all ills for the price of staying with them for three weeks. Just reading their published case studies was inspiring, though I was worldly wise enough to know that they were hardly going to point out any failures amongst their clientele. I bit the bullet, signed up and paid, and soon I was touching down at Miami International.

The Hippocrates Institute is about 120km north of Miami via those iconic beaches that you only ever see on TV. However, the Institute itself is set inland in its own spacious, tropical setting. As promised, the welcome was both warm and efficient. There was a guided tour around the facility – the Therapy Centre, Organic Salon, mineral pools, library, saunas, mini gyms, meditation yurts, juice bar, dining hall as well as my neat and comfortable accommodation.

The following morning consisted of orientation and core lectures. Then, with the help of the staff, I relaxed into the rest of my time there. There were consultations personal to each guest. Most guests had medical issues of one kind or another and the Institute promised and provided a vast range of treatments and therapies. As well as my accustomed yoga, massage and gym there was a hypobaric chamber. There were all sorts of other offerings, some of which I had never heard of and didn't get to try. There were a number of optional lectures. One of the cornerstones of the Institute is, of course, the natural and organic foods and juices. The mealtime buffets were unlimited plant-based food – vegetables, fruit, pulses as well as green juices, wheatgrass and so on.

It was a great three weeks and I felt on top of the world. Indeed the wholesome food and beneficial activities worked wonders. Sadly, once I reverted to my normal lifestyle, those benefits fell away. The co-founder of the Institute is the impressive Brian Clement who delivered several lectures during my time there. Interestingly, both he and the Institute have come under some fire for supposedly making exaggerated claims and misrepresentation.

Make your own minds up folks. I loved my time there with great benefits.

✈

I'd timed my visit to Miami to coincide with the WSCC Spinning Convention. I was by now a competent instructor but was interested to see what was new. It was well worth attending, and made me realise that I had a bit of catching up to do. My lasting memory was of 300 participants in the hall being instructed by a South African woman. Behind her, on a giant screen, was video – in this case of animals in their natural habitat, the uplifting music a perfect accompaniment to the sweating bikers. It was exciting, it was the future, and of course, video has quickly become commonplace in the world of spinning in the years since.

I left Florida with at least one tangible item for my financial outlay – a Swiss Ball instructor's certificate!

Everything has a finite life, especially as one moves through middle age. This was all very well and good, but I became restless again after three years in Mallorca. I was feeling stressed and tired. This wasn't what I wanted to do with the rest of my life. I needed another change, another challenge. But what? I hadn't a clue.

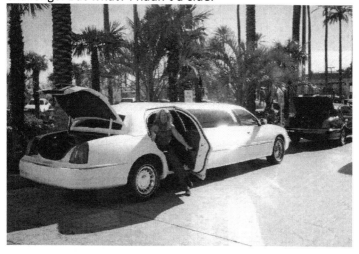

Limo in Vegas

India

Life is the combination of body, senses, mind and reincarnating soul. Ayurveda is the most sacred science of life, beneficial to humans both in this world and the world beyond.
(Charaka)

Restless, yes. Needing a challenge, yes. Not the sort of challenge that might involve rowing the Atlantic or climbing Mount Everest though. I felt I needed to explore my horizons. Years ago, those horizons were pretty limited, but now I wanted to make up for lost time and I was treading water here in Mallorca.

I was continually looking at ways, methods, techniques to make my body more comfortable. As I've mentioned, I'd more or less sworn off painkillers. In my previous life I'd have swallowed them like Smarties and accepted the mind numbness that came along with it. I was a different person now.

I'd read about Ayurveda of course, along with a host of other methods of healing. Many of these methods are super-quacky and aimed at the desperate who will part with their money in the hope and belief that their ailments will be cured. This is exploitation of the worst kind – ruthless chancers who care nothing for those who are attracted to their dubious wares. I put them in the same category as drugs dealers, feeding off human weaknesses.

Of course, there are many alternative methods and medicines. Often these work for some, not for others. They include acupuncture, hypnosis, Reiki, a host of food supplements. I'd already found benefits from practicing yoga, but Ayurveda appealed to me, not least because of its undoubted longevity, but also it gave me an excuse to be off on my travels once more.

I researched the matter more fully and decided I had much to gain and little to lose. Living in India could be done cheaply, it seemed, unless you were after Western-style comforts and luxuries.

Kerala is a state on the western Malabar Coast of India, on the Arabian Sea. It is warm to hot all the year round, though freshened by sea breezes and the plentiful rainfall and monsoons. It also seemed to be quite a centre for those wishing to seek out Ayurveda. I'd done enough research; Kerala might have been invented for me. I immediately booked a one-way ticket and left Mallorca behind, though I was destined to return later.

I arrived at Trivandrum airport, via Dubai in the middle of the night. The airport serves the city of Thiruvananthapuram, in the state of Kerala. I imagined peacefulness; the scent of exotic plants wafting on the warm breeze. I imagined a lovely, airy bed and a long, peaceful sleep.

The airport was horrendous. The terminal was packed, it was bedlam. In the main, it was women awaiting their men who make their living in Dubai. Colourful admittedly, but noisier than you can imagine. It was not exotic plants I smelt. God no, it was a dreadful stench of bodies. It was an immediate culture shock and, if I could have, I'd have turned right around and climbed back on that lovely, air-conditioned plane. I thought I was a seasoned traveller.

As an obvious Westerner with money (ha!) I was assailed on all sides.
'Taxi Miss, very quick!.'
'Water here, very cooling!'
'I take you to fine hotel, very cheap!'

I suppose I ought to have been thankful that I wasn't a man and been offered 'Lovely virgin girl, come this way sir!' In the end, just to get out of that Hades, I followed a young man, the mob lessening in number as they turned their attention to new targets. I was directed into a tuk tuk, a kind of three-wheeled motorised scooter. I was to become familiar with these over the next few weeks. 'Cheap hotel, town centre', I instructed more in hope than expectation. Any preconceptions I'd had were already dashed. I closed my eyes and let myself be transported into the city. Fortunately, the city centre was only a few miles away and my driver stopped outside an ominous-looking neon sign which blinked 'Hotel' at me, putting me in mind of a Jack Nicholson horror movie. When my driver returned and eagerly picked up my bags and beckoned me to the door, I was too weary to argue.

At least it was cheap – that much I admit. I was shown to a room by a sleepy night porter. It was horrible, dirty, toilets not working, bedclothes with dubious stains on them and goodness knows what crawling in them. I had mentioned a two-week stay to the man, but resolved there and then to find a better place the next day. In the meantime, I threw myself onto the uncomfortable bed, determined to awake strong and refreshed around 9am.

At 5am I was awakened by a cacophony out in the street. I rolled over, hoping that it would go away. No chance. It turned out that this was rush hour in downtown Thiruvananthapuram. I had headed to India looking for peace, healing, a release of stress. This was only making it worse. Later in the day I tracked down another hotel, checking out of the first though I'd stupidly booked for two weeks. I spent the next week trying to find somewhere half decent but it was a parade of dirt, ants, bugs, in one case frogs, and things not working. My big mistake was not to have pre-booked at an Ayurveda centre. After a week of bed-hopping this I finally did.

The Ayurvedic Centre

It was lovely, beautiful, clean. Anything would have been better than the fleapit hotels of Thiruvananthapuram, but it was luxury. For a while anyway I stayed there as a resident. I was treated like royalty, as indeed was everyone there. Every day a doctor assessed me and monitored my progress. There were pools, relaxation areas, massage with special oils. There were also sea swims in the nearby, warm Arabian Sea. There were three meals a day along Ayurvedic principles, with plenty of cool, refreshing water.

Ayurveda promotes balance between one's body and mind. Proper food combinations are an integral part of this based on an individual's *doshas*. Everyone has three *doshas* which are types of energy which circulate within your body. It is the balancing of these *doshas* which is crucial.

Each person's prescribed diet is therefore somewhat different, but good and wholesome non-processed foods are to the fore. Fruits, vegetables, legumes, grains, plenty of herbs and spices.

After only a short time following this regime, I was feeling much better and the relaxation and feeling of wellbeing had kicked in. I met some lovely people there too. Not all of them were sick or injured by any means. They too appreciated the benefits that Ayurveda can bring. I'd recommend it to anyone.

I couldn't really afford to pay resident rates for much longer now, so it was out with me back into cheap accommodation again. That was OK as I continued to visit the Centre as a day visitor.

The Release

One extraordinary experience that I experienced in India was the 'release' of my dead father. There was nothing premeditated about this little ceremony, but Ella, the woman I first met at the Ayurvedic centre immediately sensed something about me.

'Oh, I feel so sorry for you. He didn't mean to do it.'

'Who? Do what?'

'Your father. He didn't mean to do it.'
'My father's dead!'
'Yes, but he hasn't passed over.'

By degrees, and over coffee, I began to understand. Since I had started travelling (once I had sufficiently recovered from my accident) it felt as if I was being pulled in different directions. I wanted to do things, go places, but somehow, I'd end up doing different things, ending up in different places. What Ella was saying started to make some sense.
'Yes, your father's dead but it wasn't his time. He hasn't fully passed over. He's attached himself to you.'
'How do you mean?'
'Attached himself. You had a bad accident, fell down stairs? He wanted to take you with him.'
'But...'
'It didn't work. He's still attached to you, trying to control you.'
'He was trying to kill me?'
'Yes, but only so he could be with you. He's sorry, he didn't mean to cause you harm.'

This might explain why I didn't feel entirely in control of my destiny, but what, if anything, could I do about it? Quite how Ella knew so much I didn't try to question. There is so much that I've taken on trust since the accident and I was prepared to trust this woman, to a certain degree anyway.
'You must release him, help him to pass over. I can assist you, if you will trust me.'
'What must I do?'

'There is a temple, near here. It is a simple ceremony. I will take you.'

'OK, if you think it will help. Do we need to make an appointment?'

'It is best if you go soon. Tomorrow morning? I will drive you there. If you trust me.'

As I found out later, the Thiruvallam Parasurama Temple is the only temple in Kerala State dedicated to Lord Parasurama, the creator of Kerala, according to local legend. The temple is both ancient and impressive, some 800 years old. It is listed in India as a monument of national importance.

So, early next morning, the two of us set off. The temple itself was a few kilometres away and the traffic conditions were as you might expect from television documentaries – tuk tuks, sacred cows, bicycles, all manner of motor vehicles, people and animals jostling and beeping for right of way. An added worry, said Ella, was that my dead (but not yet passed over) father knew what was happening and would try to stop us. Fortunately, we arrived at the temple in one piece.

Ella led me into the impressive temple, spoke a few words to one of the men who seemed to be in charge. He led us through several rooms to one where a few others were gathered, sitting on the floor. I was invited to sit with them. 'Where, on this floor?' I asked.

'Yes, sit down here,' said Ella.

'But it's filthy, I can't sit here.' You could tell the person who was used to her home comforts. From somewhere, Ella produced sheets of newspaper and laid them on the ground for me. Less than grateful, I painfully plonked myself down. It was still an effort for me to perform such simple tasks, but I settled down, cross-legged, on my newspaper. Ella disappeared, to appear shortly afterwards at a nearby window. It was good of her to give me so much support.

A few more people gathered, mainly women but a few men. We were all sitting in a sort of a circle. Music and chanting drifted in from elsewhere in the temple, as did smoke and incense. Clearly there was other stuff going on elsewhere, but Ella had explained that our group were all gathered here for a common purpose. Or sort of. I can't imagine that they were all trying to release their fathers! But all had lost someone. We waited. I became conscious that everyone was scrutinising me, staring. It was disconcerting, but I was to understand that here in India there is no social taboo about staring. As the only white person in attendance, I guess I was a bit of a curiosity. I got used to this during my time in the country.

At length the priest, or pujari, made an entrance in his robes. He chanted and intoned away, though goodness knows what he was saying. Maybe the others knew. Then we were each issued with a palm leaf. I glanced at Ella in the window and she gestured that I should hold it up, as I now saw the others were doing. The priest came around to each of us, placing rice in our palm leaves with more prayers. Was this the end? Far from it. I was terribly uncomfortable sitting on the ground by this stage but resigned myself to putting up with it. More things joined the rice in our palm leaves – flowers, leaves, herbs, something that made an unpleasant pong as well.

At last the ceremony ended and people started to file out. Ella waved me to come outside, still carrying my palm leaf and contents. 'Now we must go to the river,' she said. The River Karamana was only a little walk away, down a wooded track. Other people were going that way, some bearing palm leaves like me. We reached the river. 'Now,' Ella said, 'you must go to the river edge, turn your back and throw everything over your shoulder. At the same time pray to your god that your father's soul be released and pass on.' So that is exactly what I did.

Within 24 hours I felt an incredible relief, a lightness. I can't say that I felt terribly burdened beforehand but the sensation was palpable. My father had passed over.

At no stage did anyone ask for money, or anything else, in return.

I was in India for about 10 weeks in all. At this stage the visit had served its purpose. The Ayurvedic centre had been great but I'd taken what I'd needed from it. I could put the dietary lessons into practise in other places. I started thinking of moving on once again. A friend in Mallorca had an uncle whose friend lived in Colombo, the capital of Sri Lanka. She said that she would provide an introduction should I wish to stay with him awhile.

So here I went again. With this flimsy introduction and, once more on impulse rather than as a result of planning, I was off on my travels once more.

Sri Lanka

Good ideas can also be bad choices
(Carlos Wallace)

Arrival in Colombo

Sri Lanka is only a hop across the Laccadive Sea and
Colombo, the capital, is on the west coast. My early days in
Colombo with Jerome (to whom I had been given an
introduction) and his nephew David are well documented in
my diary which I had briefly kept. Here then is a full, though
edited extract.

Arrived in Colombo to be met by David, Jerome's
nephew. Jerome was introduced to me by email from a
friend in Mallorca who thought as he was here, I could meet
up with him and maybe have some company. Oh my
goodness how wrong could I be. David, a charming and well-
mannered man (separated, in his 40s) took me to his taxi,
carrying all my luggage. We got in the car and there was an
instant likeability, I felt, on both sides. We talked about my
life briefly and also his family situation, which was obviously
very hard for him to talk about – he had two young children
who he was not allowed to visit. I felt very sorry for him and
we changed subject quickly. I then mentioned I was to meet
someone here who would be very close to me. He
straightaway said 'it is me!' I laughed. He has a good sense
of humour.

We arrived at a nice-looking apartment block in the centre of Colombo. How civilised after being in India. David rang the bell and Jerome appeared, a very short Asian-looking man with shoulders up to his neck, a very stressed looking man, very tidily dressed, but hard looking eyes. We shook hands and he invited me in and sat down. 'David, get some drinks,' he said. He introduced David as firstly his servant and secondly his nephew. 'David will take you anywhere you decide to go. I will fix everywhere for you – acupuncture, yoga, botox. I'm a fixer,' he said. 'What you need you shall get.' A man who is looked up to, I thought. I decided to take a chance on him and trust him.

He offered me his home for as long as I needed and he gave me a door key. He took me four floors higher in the lift to find a beautiful infinity pool with sun deck overlooking the city of Colombo. I could have stayed here for hours just watching and listening to life down below. He said feel free to use the pool whenever you want. My favourite pastime, so I would certainly be up at 7am to use it! Later that day Jerome took me to the local cricket club for a snack. It was beautiful, so colonial, and the staff were very friendly, although I did feel women staring at me as I arrived. I thought they probably just knew Jerome and wondered who I was (never even thinking I would be classed as a hooker)! Ordered some prawns (as I had been deprived in India because of ayurvedic treatment, no meat, no fish). Jerome just wanted a prawn or two of mine, which I didn't think anything of. He ordered a large whiskey (it was 5pm after all). I just had a water and said 'I don't drink alcohol' – he made a snide comment that I was no fun.

He asked for the bill and said 'Oh you can pay if you like'. I didn't mind as he was giving me his home, although I thought it was a bit rude to ask. Anyway we left and returned to the apartment. I was then introduced to his Chinese girlfriend called We. She was beautiful, as Jerome kept telling me, 'isn't she good for 40!' God knows what she saw in him, obviously money. That evening Jerome contacted lots of people on the phone, organising Chinese doctors for the morning, a printer to get business cards, a general supermarket for a little bit of retail therapy. As he carried on with the whiskey he got louder and louder. We had already gone to her room; she knew him better than I. David and I were flirting in the kitchen and Jerome proceeded to tell me David was his servant and he didn't think I understood this. But he's not my servant, I thought. A little bit of jealousy I felt. 'David go out and get my medicines' – he wanted him well away from me.

I decided to go to bed early and say I was tired and left him getting more drunk. 'Oh stay and talk awhile. I've been so desperate for English company. We is lovely but doesn't understand much English.'

'OK then', I said. He then started to 'cry'. Oh poor guy I thought (it was obviously the booze). I explained that I was an early bird.

'Well we are not here,' he replied.

Next morning I swam, had breakfast and wrote some emails. David was up early too and he said that he would be travelling with me for appointments. Jerome eventually surfaced with We behind him. 'We darling, why don't you go with them?' said Jerome. He was clearly suffering from a hangover, chesty cough and bad hip! We left in a taxi which David ordered. I found (what I thought was) a great acupuncturist as We spoke in Chinese to him so he knew my problems. It was painful but no pain, no gain. Then I managed to order business cards, getting discount with David's help. We then went to the market for food – I bought a fair amount to contribute. I gave David money to buy Jerome a bottle of whiskey! Expensive here but that wasn't an issue. I just wanted to pay my way. I knew whiskey would please him, never thinking he was a raging alki! We returned to the apartment with everything – Jerome was watching cricket and horse racing, making a lot of noise about who would win.

'I want to talk about a business proposal,' Jerome said 'but on a clear head, tomorrow afternoon we will talk. Today I want to show you around the hotels in Colombo, all my favourites, everyone knows me. David do you want to come?'

'No thanks.' David knew Jerome's behaviour would not be good so he used the time to be with his own friends.

We got in a taxi and We came too. Jerome started to be very rude to the driver as he did not always understand our English. We first went to the Hilton, five or six restaurants, buffet style in a beautiful setting over the lake. 'Just go and look,' he said 'we are not eating here! We will go snack at Barefoot.' Wherever that was. I really wanted to eat at the hotel, it looked scrumptious. What was a man like this looking for? Anyway, once we eventually got around a couple of the hotels 'just looking' we went to watch some jazz and had a snack. Jerome said music made him feel better when he felt down. We kept looking at me – we were bored. 'OK let's go,' he said, 'you are fed up. I need to talk to you at home.' Jerome has to be top dog, or think he is. I paid for the lunch as Jerome had no change! 'I will give you mine and We's when I have change.'

'No probs,' I said, but I was beginning to get bells ringing in my ears as he never paid for meals, just small taxi amounts.

We got back home and he said 'OK let's have a business meeting. Firstly, I have no money. My wife stole my business and my millions, but I always get back on top. Ann (ex-wife) has invested in my new venture and a few of my friends have.' He gave me letters to read, and a business plan. I had already heard of outsourcing in India (he just looked at me). He wants to outsource in Sri Lanka with solicitors and accountants, but needs backers. He wants to keep 51% and sell 49% shares. I was very wary of him.
'Where is your 51% then if you have no money?' I said
'You're not stupid, are you?' he said.
'Well I think I'm quite intelligent but I'm happy playing with MLC. (Mallorca Ladies Club)'.
'I can undercut the Indians in Sri Lanka by 40%,' he said, then giving me lots of figures which really didn't register.
'Don't decide now anyway, let me know soon though.'
'I will think about it.'
'Ann has faith in me,' he said, thinking that would convince me.

Later that evening Jerome started cooking dinner. I had bought some lovely Seer Fish (like tuna) so he was cooking and drinking at the same time. 'OK, help yourself, I will eat later.' So I served myself from the cooker. Jerome went on his computer to listen to BBC London News. He lives there some of the time. He was getting more pissed. I decided to go to my room and read as I knew Jerome would end up in a heap soon and We would have to put him to bed. He had been getting very rude with me and I felt tense.

I got up next day and went for my swim. We and I went to the Bhudda Temple. I saw the high priest and got very emotional about my accident and the pains I am left with. He got me some oil and said if I rub it on for three days I will improve. He blessed me and I put some small notes in the box. We walked around more and I was quite happy to stay for a while and ask for help quietly. We and I then walked around the lake and saw more bhuddas and prayed a little more.

We then went to the department store near the apartment and found a few nice tops and trousers and returned. David was very quietly sweeping floors and generally being the servant. He is worth so much more than that. We always exchanged smiles and gave each other loving gestures. He had touched my heart but I did not know why. I realised at this stage We was Jerome's prostitute (but was fed up of his drinking). David was just his slave and I was there to give him money for his whiskey and gambling.

I felt uneasy.

Escape from Colombo, with an accomplice

Things didn't improve between me and Jerome. When he realised that he wasn't going to get investment monies out of me he became ruder and more offensive. It was clear that my time here was coming rapidly to an end.

Poor David was treated even worse of course. Unbeknown to me, he was hatching his own plan. One day he was skivvying – sweeping, cleaning. We were alone. 'You have to get out of here,' he whispered to me, continuing to sweep.
'Why, David?'
'He is dangerous you must leave.' Then he continued 'Can I come with you?'

I was flabbergasted, but what David proposed made some sense. I couldn't stay. The plan was that David would ask Jerome if he could take me sightseeing in his car, but, unbeknown to Jerome, neither of us would return. So that was how it went. Like an eloping couple in a silent movie we secretly packed our bags and made our escape.

The car was soon abandoned and we took to the train. This was both worrisome and exciting for me. David was my willing guide but he relied on me for money. We were on the run, though it was doubtful if Jerome would be after us with a shotgun. We had taken nothing of his and owed him nothing. I was having an adventure with a nice man, though goodness knows where it would end.

We headed by train to Hikkaduwa, a beach resort about 100km south of Colombo. Once there, David found us a hotel though they had only one room. To be fair, David asked if he could share my bed. I refused, though maybe if he had pressed me on the matter... Anyway he took the rebuttal well and slept the night on the floor.

Well, Hikkaduwa isn't a place you can visit and not visit the beach. It is a popular surf spot and it was a lovely day. By this time I trusted David, though in many ways I needed to trust him. I am a good judge of character and that has rarely let me down. He therefore stood by our bags while I went for a swim. The sea was beautiful but...disaster, as I walked up the beach I felt something on my leg. Something had bitten me. I tried to take no notice but quickly my leg became very swollen. David was worried and quickly he found me a hospital.

Now, in Sri Lanka (as with India) there are government-sponsored free hospitals. Anyone can receive medical attention there. David found one nearby and rushed me there. Well, the waiting area was packed with locals screaming, shouting, crying. We walked to the desk where we were seen by a saint of a receptionist amongst the chaos.

'Did you bring your sheets and pillow?' she enquired. The answer was, of course, no. Nonetheless I was admitted and found a bed to lie on. I used my handbag as a pillow. A doctor came to examine me and to take a blood sample, but by this time I was freaked with the noise and everything. I refused to let him take a blood sample. Here was I, a privileged white woman, turning down what was no doubt perfectly good medical care just because it was free. Instead I begged David to take me to a private hospital.

What a trooper David was. He could have abandoned me to my fate, but of course, I had the money. He sought out a private hospital even though I didn't have medical insurance. What a horrible, long journey by tuk tuk. I was feeling wretched and sick by now, my leg like a balloon, but eventually we arrived and I was swiftly admitted.

I was there for five days. I really had been badly poisoned. In the end they needed to cut out the poison. Despite the mounting expense, I had a lovely room and the stress I'd felt just fell away. In the meantime I had no option but to trust David with my credit and debit cards, to draw money, to buy food, to find his own accommodation. He never let me down.

My doctor at the hospital befriended me, took to chatting to me. He took a dim view of David hanging around and started warning me about him. Poor David had done nothing to make me mistrust him. However, the doctor now confided in me that he was to open an Ayurvedic centre in nearby Galle and he offered to take me there to stay. No charge. So off I went with the doc, telling David where I was going and making sure he had enough money to be getting on with.

I ought to have known. I was old enough now but I was still acting on impulse rather than thinking things out. Driving to Galle the doc's hand wandered over to my knee. After I'd pushed it away a few times he protested.

'No sorry, friendship only. Understand?'
He laughed. 'It is different maybe in your country but here in Sri Lanka men have many women.'

We got to Galle, and indeed there was a clinic, though it was unfinished. I had my own room, lockable, and it was all very nice. I stayed there for a number of days, despite, every night, having to ignore a quiet knocking on my door. There were massages by day by female staff, there were baths with rose petals. It was all very nice for the time being.

Maybe I'd have been there to this day, who knows, but now there was a louder knocking. It was David who had been lurking nearby. He urged me to leave. Although I was happy and relaxed, I knew David better by now than to ignore what he was saying. We chatted.
'David, I think I'll go back to India for a while, maybe to the Centre there. Then I'll head back to Mallorca.'
'OK. Can I come with you?'
'What? To Mallorca?'
'Yes.'

I agreed. He could come to Mallorca and join me in a couple of weeks. I had to agree to pay his fare. He had no money of his own. Again I trusted him with my credit card and away he went and bought us both air tickets – Colombo to Mallorca. I left a big suitcase with him, including a big Bhudda I'd bought on impulse.

David accompanied me to Colombo airport. He gave me the date and time of his arrival in Mallorca a couple of weeks later.

Back in Mallorca, I went to meet his flight. He wasn't on it. I didn't hear from him until a year later. He then tried to phone me without success. Then I got an email. Jerome had caught up with him and had had him thrown into jail on some pretext or other. He asked me could he still come to Mallorca. I said yes, but he would need to pay for his own ticket this time, and he could bring my suitcase.

I'm still waiting.

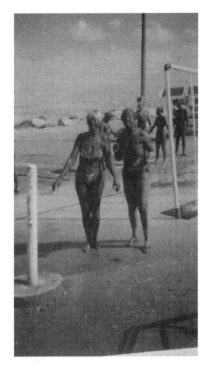

Sandi & Jean, Dead Sea 2002

Marbella (Malaga)

I pass this way one time only
A fleeting minute in eternity
And what I do in that minute
Is entirely up to me
(David Harris)

My time in Mallorca, via India and Sri Lanka, had come to a natural end. It seems as if I live my life in mini-bites, welcoming in new opportunities yet knowing instinctively when their time is up and new adventures beckon. I had a hankering to return to Malaga where I'd spent a couple of happy years.

I'd sold my caravan in Fuengirola to a German girl before I'd left for Mallorca. In any case I wanted to start afresh, though in a part of the world which I knew suited me well and with which I was reasonably familiar. Marbella is a little further south than Fuengirola and I got myself a nice flat in Marbella Old Town. Bit by bit, I settled in. I joined the nearby gym – always a factor now in choosing a place to live. It was cheap and I would go there every day to use the gym and the pool.

Marbella has an ancient history and archaeological heritage, but it is these days a city of 140,000 inhabitants and is, of course, an international tourist centre, but teeming cities all have their 'villages' and, one by one, I started to catch up with old friends. Others had gone, of course. And, almost inevitably, I started up my networking activities again. This time it was Costa Business Club, bringing business people together in social surroundings. It wasn't dissimilar to the Mallorca Ladies Club, but bringing men into the fold. It was fun. Lunches, chats, a chance for people to get to know one another but with no pressures.

One lovely person I met was Gilly Jaxson. Gilly was a fabulous singer and used to entertain audiences at the beach, in bars, in clubs. She was also a healthy living advocate and, into the bargain, was a clairvoyant. I'm in my element with clairvoyants, and one day she told my fortune. Looking closely until she was sure, she told me that she saw a very big house, and that I would live there.

I thought little more of it then but, in truth, little clouds of doubt were forming about my decision to return to Malaga. Yes I was happy enough, but wasn't I just repeating a part of a life I'd lived previously? Most people would count themselves lucky to be in my position, that much is true. Since the accident it seemed that I needed to do so much more than cruise along comfortably, albeit still with a constant level of residual pain which I was constantly trying to ease.

Gilly left to go and live and work in Tenerife. She invited me over. As it so happened, Bryan, the faith healer from the caravan site, and his wife Sheila, had since located to Tenerife as well. The stars were in alignment. After just six months in Marbella I prepared to leave for a second time.

Tenerife

*Wheels are made for rolling, mules are made to
pack
I've never seen a sight that didn't look better looking back
(Lerner & Loewe)*

Goodbyes and hellos

I'm not good at goodbyes. I don't do leaving parties. I get
upset. In this, the second (post-accident) phase of my life
I've become something of a drifter. Tentative roots are
tugged loose and I'm off again once I get the mind to go.

So, I piled the Escort high with my essential
belongings. My faithful blue Escort went everywhere with
me. Richard's old banger, a Renault, came in handy for non-
essentials. I drove the Renault to a compound near to the
airport to await collection sometime in the future.

Off I set for the port of Cadiz. Despite my
experience of travelling I'm still not the most confident
driver, especially when I'm on my own. I panic unreasonably
about getting lost. I mean, how lost can you get travelling
from A to B along well-signposted roads? I worry about
driving on the right, though I know I am perfectly capable.
Once I get attuned to the roads the only real concern I have
is filtering onto main roads to the left. Even now I have
limited motion in my neck so turning my head owl-like to
judge the oncoming traffic isn't an option. Thank goodness
cars have mirrors, and the journey was uneventful.

The border town of Tarifa might have been a distraction, but it was familiar to me. At that time they used to run bus trips down to Gibraltar from the Fuengirola area. It was a popular thing to do for a bit of sightseeing and shopping, especially for the Brits. I believe these days the Spanish authorities aren't so amenable to all and sundry sauntering backwards and forwards across the border.

I arrived at Cadiz where I was to catch the ferry down to Tenerife. I stopped for the night in a guest house and set off for the ferry the next morning. I'd booked with the company *Armas* for reasons of economy. It was a freighter, mainly used by lorry drivers delivering goods to and from the Canaries. A luxury liner it was not, and to be fair I didn't expect it to be. On the plus side I had my own cabin. Not what a queen would have accepted, but I was travelling cheap and it was quite all right for me. Too bad if it hadn't been all right. I spent most of the 48-hour voyage in it, mainly because there was little else to do. A tip to adventurous folk wishing to travel on the cheap. Search around for those freight companies that offer passage to foot passengers. You can find some real bargains. OK admittedly you might end up in one or two strange places, and behind schedule, but you'll eat heartily and be made very welcome.

No luxury dining room, dressing for dinner or sitting at the captain's table. Meals were served in what was basically a works canteen. I'd eat up and head back to my cabin. As the WiFi was hopeless, and I'm not much of a reader, this made for a long and wearisome journey. As seems to come naturally to me, I did bump into a chap by the name of Bernd. He was a German and bodybuilding was his 'thing'. His claim to fame is that he was big mates with Arnold Schwarzenegger, a fellow bodybuilder and former governor of California. 'Arnie' was usually referenced in our conversations. A nice guy though. I bumped into him later in a gym in Tenerife and I'm still in contact with him.

I was to repeat this sea journey three months later, flying back to Malaga to bring Richard's Renault back.

Mercifully, the main port of Tenerife, and its capital Santa Cruz, is the first bit of the island that the Cadiz boat reaches. Tenerife itself is the largest of the Canary Islands, the others being Fuerteventura, Gran Canaria, Lanzarote, La Palma, La Gomera and El Hierro. Its most recognisable feature is the volcanic Teide which attracts many visitors. Most tourists will fly into Tenerife South, adjacent to the popular resorts, Playa de Las Americas chief amongst them. Tenerife North is notorious for being the scene of the deadliest accident in aviation history when, in 1977, two Boeing 747s collided on the runway, killing 583 people.

It was south I headed. The 80km drive is easy – the main road snakes around the coastline of much of the island and you just need to point the car in the right direction and concentrate. My destination was Adeje, which is north of Los Cristianos and Playa de las Americas. My immediate mission, to hook up again with Gilly, and this I did. She was living in a little cottage on the beach at Salvaje. It was nice to catch up though Gilly hadn't really settled into Tenerife life. Her prime source of income was her singing. She was finding it tough to attract paying audiences. Before long she took the decision to head back to Malaga which saddened me somewhat, but I had no thoughts about returning with her. Gilly met an Australian guy after returning to Malaga and now lives with him in Australia.

After a couple of days in a guest house I started to look for a little apartment to rent. I stayed a week in La Caleta, near the beach. It was noisy, and I preferred to live somewhere a bit quieter. The little town of Adeje is a little inland, at the foot of the mountains which rise towards the centre of the island. It is quiet, picturesque, and retains the feel of the 'real' Spain, though still popular with visitors for those reasons. I asked around, fancying living there for a while. And I was lucky enough to bump into a woman called Sarah who told me an apartment next to hers was to let. Access to a swimming pool too. A gym close by, which I really couldn't do without. It ticked enough boxes for me and I moved in.

There I spent my first couple of months, generally finding my feet, settling in. I went to the gym, sorted out the flat, met a few people, improved my poor spoken Spanish. Everywhere in Spain you can make yourself understood in English. The people are well used to the lazy Brits at this stage, but it's always better if you can have at least a halting conversation with the local people.

At which point I must make a confession. Booze had led to my downfall, and it was a long time after my accident before I touched another drop. But in Spain a glass of wine, sangria, it was part of the way of life. In Malaga I began to worry that, although I wasn't drinking a great deal, I often fancied a little drink. So much so that I took myself along to a local branch of AA. I was amazed. It wasn't what I expected at all. What's more, I made instant friends! So now, here in Tenerife, I found myself getting a little depressed. Was there a causal link with my drinking? After my previous positive experience, I trotted along to the Los Cristianos branch, a little way the other side of Las Americas. I wasn't disappointed. Again, they were a lovely group of people, not a bit gloomy like you might expect. It helped deal with what may have become a major issue.

As you'll know by this time, I love meeting new people. Amongst those I met was a woman called Linda. She was certainly unconventional. Linda had a lovely disposition and gave the impression that she had no worries. You only had to do the right things and wonderful things would happen. Though, as I was to find out, we all have our worries, even Linda.

However, as it happened, me and Linda got to talking about yoga retreats. Little did I suspect at first that this was to lead to something big. Yoga retreats were something we both knew something about. Suddenly we were asking each other – how about setting up a yoga retreat, here, in Tenerife? Well, naturally I was interested. After the Ladies Club in Mallorca, the Singles Club, the Costa Business Club, I was confident I could organise things. Making something that would pay, a commercial venture, was another matter. Anything along those lines I'd only ever done for a bit of fun really. I didn't lose money at it, but I had no ambitions to build a business empire.

The idea wouldn't go away. We kept meeting up, for coffee, for tapas. We talked of other stuff but it came back to the same subject. One day we saw a classified advertisement in the local paper. Large property to let. It was here, in Adeje though not in the town. We called the number given and spoke to the owner. Could we view the place? 'Meet me at the petrol station in Armeñime,' he said. A good job he guided us there. We followed him up hills, through woods, and eventually we found it. It was a banana plantation! The house was huge. It was exactly what Gilly had seen in my future! It gave me goosebumps, and I was immediately inclined to take it on sight.

The owner had come down from Santa Cruz. He immediately buttered us up by saying that he liked us and was willing to rent to us. 'Which bit is for rent?' asked Linda. 'All of it,' said the owner. This we never expected. We'd originally envisaged a couple of rooms or so.
'How much?' we asked, certain that it would be out of our league.
'700 Euros. A month. Including services. Would that be ok?'

700 Euros. 350 each, services included. It was nothing. Well, not nothing but it didn't take us long to decide. Even by our 'back of a fag packet' calculations we were sure it was affordable. Living at the plantation (shortly to be renamed *Refugio Plantacion*) we would save paying rent at our present flats, plus whatever we might make from running classes and other events. Not that I ever went into these various ventures hoping, or indeed expecting, to make money. I didn't wish to lose money either, but

meeting people, networking, offering a service that I enjoyed myself, well that was enough for me.

Then, a blow. Linda got cold feet. Having slept on the matter, or rather not sleeping but worrying, she decided the whole project was too much for her. Not so much the cost but the work involved, the responsibility of working as one of a partnership. She was abjectly apologetic but said that she had to pull out of the deal. I was upset.

What was I to do? If Gilly had still been here in Tenerife then she may have provided the solution, but she wasn't. The easiest thing to do would have been to pull out of the deal. A stream always runs downhill, seeking the path of least resistance. At one time I might have done likewise, but I had changed. I was up for challenges now. Not challenges of the sky diving or mountaineering sort. My damaged body wouldn't have allowed me even if I was of that persuasion. I knew I could organise, I was good with people (NFH apart) and I now had some knowledge and experience of yoga, and yoga retreats, though I had yet to teach the subject.

In short, I signed the lease. It was mine. It was June 2012.

Refugio Plantacion Tenerife

The building itself was just idyllic. It had originally been a family home. I never learnt the history but it was quite likely built and owned by a rich Englishman in the days when England colonised half of the world. In more recent times this had been a working banana plantation and the building had housed the plantation workers. The plantation manager had lived there until recently and he still lived nearby and kept an eye on things generally. It was huge – four double bedrooms, a big lounge, a serviceable kitchen and other rooms. Much bigger than I had envisaged but who knew what I might make of it.

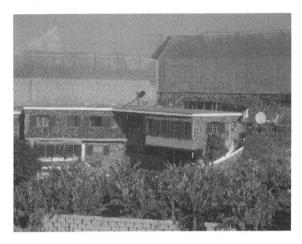

Refugio Plantacion Retreat

It was scary at first. It was so quiet and I've never been a fan of darkness. I got used to it in time. There was little by way of furniture or effects in the house, so I activated my inner shopper. I scouted around Adeje, Las Americas and Los Cristianos to acquire what I needed to set the business up. Beds, fitted kitchen, bathroom were already in situ. I needed bedding, chairs, tables, music centre, various bits and pieces. Most of it second-hand, none of it expensive but clean and serviceable. Bikes for spinning I got free from the gym – they were throwing them out. Where necessary I got the sellers to deliver. For example, the room most suitable for yoga needed little else. I started talking to people – that I have no problem with, though on occasion it has caused me problems. First, I talked to yoga teachers and suchlike. Would they come and teach classes for me? Laura, for one example. There was Antonello, a massage therapist. I was in business.

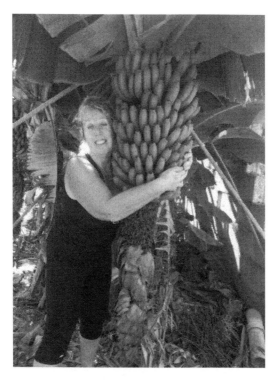

At the Refugio

I advertised. Mainly on Facebook. I continued to talk and spread the word about my little venture. Facebook is a perfect vehicle with its ripple effect. Soon numbers picked up. Yoga, massage to start with, but then I started to up my game. At this stage I should introduce Elaine Clark who was to become my rock. Elaine lived in El Medano with her husband. El Medano is about 25km away from Adeje but, notwithstanding this, she became a great help, which I was honestly beginning to need as we expanded. Elaine was a massage therapist and we met up after she contacted me via the Refugio's Facebook page. She quickly became a regular at our yoga sessions, and later when we began to offer weekly lunches. She was an unfailing source of support and advice and we were to become, and remain, firm friends.

Elaine says, 'I met Sandi about seven years ago. I came across her venture in a banana plantation on Facebook and I decided to check it out. It was a wonderful venture for her and I got on well with Sandi. I starting doing holistic massage treatments every Monday. She ran the Monday Club, like-minded people meeting up for vegan lunch and various treatments and yoga in the evening with Emily, accompanied by two lovely cats. All by donation only. It was wonderful for a while, meeting many wonderful people from all over the world who had so many things in common. 'Peace Seekers'.

'Sandi grew all her own herbs and vegetables. She was a huge fan of hemp plants and wheat grass and was always growing new and wonderful herbs such as moringa, and many I had never heard of. I learnt a lot from Sandi and her guests. She ran some fun retreats for those looking to escape the hustle & bustle of modern life. I was very impressed with her strong determination to give the project a go. I was happy to help her succeed as the whole project was rather unique and hidden away. Many people visited from far and wide. She hosted various events such as gong and cymbals nights, yoga nights, healing with energy days with some of the very best in their field. Various meditation practices, Reiki, tai chi but name but a few. It really was wonderful.

'I admired Sandi. At night time when everyone had gone home, she would stay there alone, surrounded by hunting dogs and various sounds through the night. I do remember her saying she felt a bit spooked, but she continued to keep positive with her amazing project. We had such fun and learnt so many spiritual practices. When she said that she was leaving, it was very sad after all the work she had put in. However, due to the landlord and workers on the plantation she was no longer able to continue.

'I know Sandi continued her projects elsewhere after leaving Tenerife. We continue to be in touch. She always keeps positive and enthusiastic and always has a project on the go despite life's knocks.'

From time to time we offered professional cycling training, meditation, self-empowerment, addiction recovery, other alternative therapies.

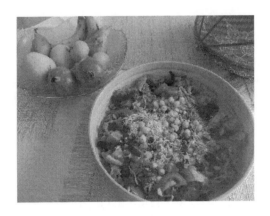

As regards the cycle training, I was seeing more and more of Richard these days. He would come and visit whenever he could, and was experienced enough now to lead groups. Tenerife is physically defined by the volcanic Mount Teide, which at 12,198 ft, is the highest point in Spain. The rest of the island, including of course the fabulous beaches, is arranged around Teide. So, and as you can imagine, the training never consisted of an easy spin along flat roads.

André and Debs, together with my 6-month-old grand-daughter Evie, also came to stay at the Refugio, which was great.

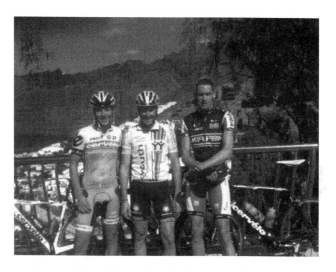

Stephen Haley, Richard, Sean Twohig at Los Gigantes

I was lucky enough to encounter Peter who lived in nearby Playa Paraiso. He became my odd-job man, maintenance man, gopher. I don't know how I'd have coped without him.

After a little while, I met a couple who walked in the area and I would often join them. We would say hello to a friendly Polish guy who was living rough, Martin. After I'd mentioned to the couple that I could do with another pair of hands they suggested that Martin might be amenable to helping out. What a good call that was. Martin became part of the staff. Peter had already built a perfect bamboo cabin for massage purposes. Now he built a similar one for Martin to sleep in. Both cabins were covered with banana leaves which were perfect for shielding them from the worst of the sun's rays.

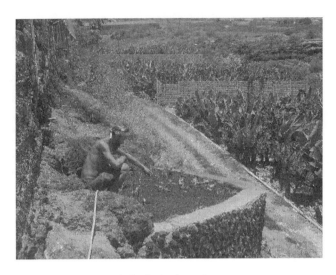

Martin in the herb garden

Martin's great achievement was building a compost toilet! Other than that, his speciality was the herb garden, which he loved. He was always happy to help out with whatever needed doing.

We had access to bananas and mangoes from the plantation. We started offering weekly lunches, speciality banana cake! This was me reprising my Ladies Club idea which I knew worked well. Would you like a sugar-free banana cake recipe, dear reader? OK, but it's very complicated.

Banana Cake
3 mashed bananas (ripe)
1/3 cup apple sauce
2 cups oats

¼ cup almond milk
½ cup raisins (optional)
1 tsp vanilla
1 tsp cinnamon

Bake at 350 for 15 – 20 minutes

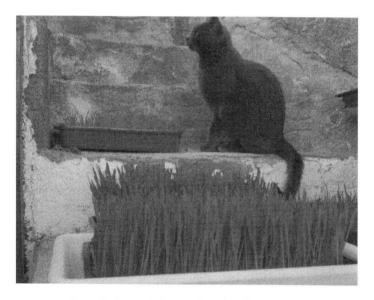

The Refugio cat Sheba guarding the wheatgrass

     We made a virtue of the freshness of our natural foods. Our fruit, veg, and herbs we either grew on site or obtained from the local market. We had fresh eggs every day. There was home grown wheatgrass. I even experimented with making my own natural products – aloe vera drink, coconut & mint toothpaste, hemp body scrub, aloe facial moisturiser. As mentioned previously, I've had an occasional issue with cancerous carcinomas. I concocted an organic lotion which really did seem to help.

We offered virtually everything from time to time. In addition to those activities already mentioned we had tarot readings, emotional freedom techniques, Chinese medicine & acupuncture, reflexology. Agatha offered gong healing, often known as gong bathing. This is a form of meditation during which varying gong vibrations are absorbed into the inner body producing relaxation, daydreams, associative thinking and animated imagination. This can only be done successfully where there is space, away from built-up areas.

The inaccessibility of the place I turned into a virtue. You won't find it on a map. It is totally secluded on the west of the mountains. Neither are there signposts. If you booked you got directions. There was a private entrance for those wishing to visit anonymously.

One day a girl in Las Americas asked me if I offered residential breaks – retreats, such as I had experienced in India. No I didn't, but I soon introduced them. It was a no-brainer. Soon these breaks were proving popular. We were a strictly no-alcohol establishment and I found that people were happy to have an enforced break from the drinking culture that tends to be the norm in Spanish beach resorts. Not so much the locals but the Brit expats and holidaymakers. The cheap local beers and lagers, deliciously cool and flavourful in the hot climate, are irresistible to many.

Back in my running days I'd met my future friend in Dawn Wheeler. I was delighted when she contacted me and came to visit the Refugio.

Dawn says, 'I was at a low ebb. I'd had a really bad time in my personal life. Then one day I was scanning through Gallery magazine and I did a double take. There was an article all about Sandi, her accident, and how she'd rebuilt her life. Well I got in contact with her and the next thing, there I was, at the plantation. It was just what I needed by way of therapy. I just floated around, did a few classes, helped out a little around the place. Sandi was so laid back. All my troubles seemed to melt away. I went back a second time and found my feet again and was ready to face the world once more.'

A woman of substances?

I still needed the pain relief that I got from regular massage. Daniel, a Spanish guy with dreadlocks, gave the best massages ever. Little did I guess why, to begin with. Cannabis in the massage cream was the answer. What a difference it made. I started to tentatively research the subject. I had no intention of starting to smoke joints or anything – I had stopped smoking many years previously. If it had a beneficial medicinal effect then I was up for trying it. I dislike conventional pain relief which always leaves me dopey and drowsy.

Recreational drugs in general have had a bad press. This is, in part, a cultural thing. In the Swinging Sixties, cannabis and LSD became synonymous with what the establishment saw as decadent and permissive behaviour by young people. Gurus such as Timothy Leary and the Maharishi Yogi preached the benefits of enlightenment if you took these substances. As those young people themselves have become part of the establishment, then the perception has become less shocking. However, the present-day fear is that relatively benign recreational drugs can lead on to 'harder' addictive drugs such as heroin and crack cocaine, which can have a devastating effect on the individual, their families and society in general. This is the reason why 'soft' drugs such as cannabis remain restricted as best, illegal at worst.

Anyway, I got to know Daniel well. He started bringing his friends to our lunches, often playing his didgeridoo. The place was beginning to have a life of its own. One day Daniel said 'This would be a great place to grow cannabis.' I suppose I must have gasped, I forget. By now I knew that cannabis could be useful in pain relief, but I had not seriously thought to try anything of that sort so far.

Medicinal cannabis i.e. the substance with the psychoactive THC removed, has become guardedly accepted as having real benefits though – certainly in Jersey – GPs are still reluctant to prescribe it. It is high time that those with the power to make decisions realise that there is a huge difference between the recreational drug and the medicinal drug. Many people in great need are being denied the latter.

So I learnt from Daniel that there was a 'Grow Shop' in Los Cristianos. Off I went, bold as brass, and bought cannabis seeds. I planted them on top of the building. Now,

Spanish law allows one to grow no more than five cannabis plants for personal usage. I'm admitting nothing but I may have accidently planted more than five. I was never any good at maths. They grew beautifully – the climate was ideal. Once the plants were ready, I took them to a room downstairs. I placed them on nylon sheets to dry out. In damper climates you'd need heaters but here in Tenerife they dried out perfectly. When ready I concocted my potion, a mixture of coconut oil and cannabis leaves. I'd boil it all up for about five hours. Then I'd mash it until it was totally gloopy. And into jars it went to be stored.

I felt very odd, high, during the manufacturing process, but that was OK. There was no one around. Now Daniel could use it when he came to do his wonderful massages. In addition, I used it to help me sleep. Just rubbed it into my skin. What a difference this would have made years earlier.

There was (probably still is) a Cannabis Club in Tenerife. I used to go there on occasion. The police tolerated it with something of a jaundiced eye but it made sense really. In cities, for example, there are one or two notorious pubs which are nothing but trouble. Troublemakers gravitate to them. The police are content to have the troublemakers contained in one place and therefore give latitude to the landlords to keep it that way. The Cannabis Club was a peaceful place and it was probably better for everyone to leave it be rather that act heavy handed and have it go underground

I finish this section with a precautionary tale. I still attended the local hospital for treatment on occasion. I must have been less than careful in cleaning out the blender after using it for my mixture, and had used it subsequently for my morning smoothie. So, I was driving to the hospital in Las Americas one day and, suddenly, I got very high. I could barely control the car and was sure that I was going to crash, but I couldn't stop in the middle of the road. Fortunately, there wasn't far to go to the hospital and, by a miracle, I escaped unscathed. I sat there for hours until the effects wore off and it was safe to move. So boys and girls, always clean your cannabis blender thoroughly.

Down on the Farm

I started hearing animal noises. No, I wasn't high or hallucinating, as you may have thought after the section above. Maybe the noises had been there all the time but I'd filtered them out. In the quiet of the evening, or in the early morning, the noises were quite audible. What sort of animals? I didn't know. I know what cats and dogs sound like – it wasn't cats or dogs. I know what noise sheep and cows make – it wasn't them. The noises seemed to be coming from somewhere below the plantation, on the lower slopes. At first, I'd simply acknowledge the sounds and dismiss them. One day – it must have been a quiet one – I decided to investigate.

I jumped in my car and headed down the narrow lanes. It didn't take me long to find the source of the strange sounds. There, behind a wire fence, were the culprits. Llamas, goats, camels, a few of each. A donkey, a few rabbits. The poor things were, in the main, lying down and showing little interest in doing anything else. The sun was, as always, shining and the animals had no shade whatsoever. Now I'm no expert but I think animals need a choice of whether or not to lie in the sun. Giving them no choice told me that no one was looking after them properly. I investigated further, and came upon a little café. I tried out my Spanglish on the woman behind the counter.

'Hola.'

'Hola. I was just wondering, whose animals are those over in the field? Who do they belong to?'

'The animals? Oh yes, those animals. They belong to my son.'

'Is your son here? Could I talk to him?'

'No he is not here. He lives in Adeje.'

'Oh. I was just wondering. Do they have enough to eat? Enough water?'

'Yes of course. All the leftovers from the café. They are fine.'

'OK. Do you mind if people, customers, feed them?'

'No, they like that.'

'It is OK if I bring them food now and again? I live just up the hill.'

'Yes of course, if you wish, but they are fine.'

It was clear that the animals were not 'fine', but I have found that not all Spanish people treat their pets and animals well. Here in Britain, people are generally caring towards their pets and know how to care for them. For example, too many dogs in Spain are tied up for hours and, lacking friendly company, become angry and vicious. It was clear that here, behind the café, nobody much cared if these animals were sick or hungry. I decided to reach out to them. So I began to visit daily. Bananas on the ground at the plantation were plentiful and free. I'd buy carrots from the local market. The animals nearly took my hand off! They happily munched away at everything I brought for them. Water too, they clearly didn't have enough. The camels wore a sort of muzzle and I would feed them carrots through the opening.

After a few days the animals were perkier, walking about, less sleepy. Soon they would hear me coming and would make a beeline towards the fence, eager to see what I'd brought for them today. It was very little work for me and it was lovely to see my new friends respond so well. Really, if we as humans make a decision to keep and cage animals it is our responsibility to ensure that they have the basics to comfortably survive.

There were sad moments too. I'd noticed one of the two snowy-white llamas had developed a bad eye, and it seemed to be getting worse. It was hardly my place to go to the café with this information. Where would it stop? One day I arrived and there was only one llama.

Antigua – Weddings and Crossroads

Back in my Mallorca days I had a friend, Debs. She is still a friend, but she is now my daughter-in-law. Of course, she's much younger than I am. I first met her parents who owned a dive school in Mallorca and it was in their shop that I first said 'Hi' to Debs. Hearing that I taught spinning classes at the local gym, Debs turned up one afternoon. We hit it off and we soon became friends.

André and Richard came to Mallorca to celebrate Richard's 21st with me, which was a lovely gesture. It was decided that we'd all go off to a local Indian restaurant. Debs and her parents came along too, so there were six of us in the party. Destiny moves in strange ways. André sat opposite Debs and, by the end of the evening there were clearly the first sparks of something special. That something special developed, and before long the new couple had moved in to live with Debs' parents.

Andre says 'The evening of Richard's 21st party was amazing. It took on a life of its own with the DJ, the laughing and dancing. The whole place joined in. I'm sure the restaurant staff are talking about it to this day.

'It was the first time I'd met Debbie. It took us all of two seconds to connect. Love at first sight may be a cliché but in our case it was absolutely true.'

After a time, they decided to travel. New Zealand was their destination and Debs began a three-year course in acupuncture. Then Debs' parents decided to move to Antigua. Debs and André joined them for a while after Debs had gained her qualification.

By this time I was living at the Refugio and one morning I received a wedding invitation! Delighted, off I went to Antigua leaving the Refugio in the hands of my trusted helpers. I stayed with friends of Debs' parents who were originally from Phoenix, Arizona. She was the sporty type and he was manager of the local Burger King. The wedding was one of the happiest days of my life to see my eldest son and his sweetheart, my friend, married there on the beach. Richard was there too, with his girlfriend.

My ex-husband Dick was there too with his partner. After the wedding (fortunately) the pair of us ended up having little mishaps. Somehow, I contracted an eye infection, and Dick fell downstairs, injuring himself. No great harm done in either case.

> *André says 'The day of our wedding was brilliant. It was picture book, barefoot on the beach in the sunshine. It was otherwise quite hard work – the days beforehand were a series of airport runs, meeting our family and other guests. Then Mum developed an eye infection, Richard fell off his bike, Dad fell down some stairs, Laura had an allergic reaction. Then afterwards the airport runs again. But yeah, it was great!'*

In 1936 the American bluesman Robert Johnson recorded a song called *Cross Road Blues*. The lyrics have often been interpreted as Johnson selling his soul to the Devil. Thirty years later a band called Cream took the song, added virtuoso rock guitar and driving bass rhythm and drums to make *Crossroads* one of their signature numbers. Guitarist Eric Clapton is the only one of the three band members living today.

Clapton is, of course, one of the world's best proponents of guitar. (Rolling Stone magazine has him second only to Jimi Hendrix.) The demons of drugs and alcohol, driven by troubled personal relationships, once took him to the brink. In his autobiography he says *'In the lowest moments of my life, the only reason I didn't commit suicide was that I knew I wouldn't be able to drink any more if I was dead. It was the only thing I thought was worth living for, and the idea that people were about to try and remove me from alcohol was so terrible that I drank and drank and drank, and they had to practically carry me into the clinic.'*

Whilst I was in Antigua I had the honour of visiting Eric Clapton's Crossroads Centre. Clapton founded this addiction and recovery centre in 1998 and has supported it financially ever since. I find it hard to believe that there is a better facility anywhere else in the world. Set next to the beach under the sunny skies, Crossroads is the ultimate. As mentioned before, I stayed with friends of Debs' parents. It was through them that I got friendly with another woman who was 'in recovery'. (I should probably clarify here that an alcoholic under treatment is permanently 'in recovery', no matter if they haven't had a drink for 20 years.) We got talking. She invited me to a meeting, a sort of AA thing. This took place at Shirley Heights. This is a former military lookout with the most amazing views. I met some wonderful people there. The Americans love our English accent.

She worked at Crossroads as a counsellor. After the Shirley Heights meeting, she asked me if I would like to take a visit, have a look around. Of course I would! The opportunity isn't afforded to many and I was honoured. My new friend vouched for me, and my back story no doubt helped. I had to sign all sorts of non-disclosure agreements.

It is vital of course that anyone undergoing treatment there (or anywhere like it) can do so with confidence that their privacy will be respected.

Although I was only a visitor on this occasion it is easy to understand how a month spent here would give you a fighting chance of getting clean and staying clean and sober. The facilities looked wonderful, complementing the idyllic setting near the beach under cloudless skies. Madly expensive no doubt, but I understand they do try to assist those of limited means where they can. Certainly it was Clapton's original intention to assist those unable to afford such treatment. It was a heart-lifting experience.

My Antigua trip was all a bit of a whirl. With a bit of jet lag thrown in, maybe I didn't appreciate the island as much as I might have. I did spend time each day in swimming off the wonderful beaches – this version of aqua-therapy continues to be wonderful for dealing with pain. So back to Tenerife and the Refugio.

On the Road Again

Of course, I ought to have put the Refugio on a proper legal footing. It had gone well past the hobby stage. However, the time never seemed right and I never got around to it. Perhaps if the Refugio had been mine, perhaps if I'd had a pushy business partner, then I might have built the business up into something meaningful. As it was, I saw this lifestyle as part of my recuperation. 'Recuperation My Lifestyle' became a catchphrase. It was being paid for by others, though I never sought to make a profit. Naturally I got all my classes free. Renew/relax/recuperate. This was what I needed and what I offered to others. It was good.

So why am I not still there?

This cycle of putting shallow roots down before moving on was becoming familiar. My mother was Irish and, though I don't know much about her family history, I'm convinced that her ancestors must have been travelling folk. Nomadic people, they might originally have moved continuously with their herds. Later, and within living memory, they would move from town to town making and mending pots and pans, horse harnesses and the like. Maybe I have a touch of nomad.

Also, the plantation manager was becoming a pest. Before I arrived, he used to live there so I always thought his nose had been put out of joint a little. Apart from attending to basic duties, he had bothered me little. This changed. He took to patrolling at night with his dogs. I quite understood that he was in charge of security, but nothing had changed since I'd been there. The plantation was quiet and peaceful at night. His changed behaviour worried me, and it was also disturbing for any overnight guests.

Something else happened. I'd bought six chickens and Martin used to look after them, bring me the eggs and so on. One morning the chicken run was damaged and all the chickens dead. Clearly an animal (a fox?) had got in. Maybe it was a coincidence, but it was another little thing that nagged away at me.

I decided not to renew the lease. By this time Martin had left anyway. He'd got himself a good job and left, leaving me with little support. I told Peter of my decision and asked him to remove the bamboo huts that he'd so cleverly constructed. He kept the dead chickens and was to move on quite unaffected by it all. He was a free spirit.

I've never been back to the Refugio. Elaine tells me that it's still all closed up.

Fuerteventura and Ibiza

I can't wait to get on the road again
Goin' places that I've never been
Seein' things that I may never see again
(Willie Nelson)

Richard helped me to pack. It was much the same story as before, loading the long-suffering Escort and Richard's Renault and leaving them at the secure car park near to the airport. Then we packed two more boxes to take with us back to Jersey. Amongst all the useful stuff were several large, prickly plants which I'd bought locally. I was reluctant to leave them behind, so we wrapped them carefully and brought them back with us. Me and Richard flew back to Jersey with the boxes. The prickly plants came to live with us at Richard's house in St Saviour. (By this time, I'd let Maggie's flat go and I'd stay with Richard whenever I came back.)

So had my wandering days come to a halt? Far from it. Though I still regarded Jersey as my home the reasons that had led me away to southern climes still remained. My body and mind still needed the warmth of the sun's healing rays. It was unsurprising when the Brit holidaymakers started bypassing Jersey for guaranteed sunshine in the 1980s. Yes, Jersey has sunshine but not enough, and the winter and spring weather can be miserable. Then came the cheap flights direct to the Med and elsewhere. Jersey's tourist industry declined. Those bleak days following my accident spent virtually immobile looking out of my lounge window at the clouds and rain still haunted me.

Another reason for the decline in Jersey's tourism industry was of course, price. The finance industry has pushed the cost of living relentlessly upwards and Jersey can no longer compete on price. Even were there to be wall-to-wall sunshine the days of Jersey as a cheap destination are long gone.

So there I was again, scanning the atlas and airline timetables. I spoke to Elaine who was still living in Tenerife. I'd been to Fuerteventura, another of the Canary Islands, at one time and I'd enjoyed my stay. Maybe me and Elaine could have a little holiday there and catch up? So it was arranged. I met her at El Mattoral Airport and we travelled north to Corralejo, a distance of about 30km. The town of Corralejo is on the northern tip of the island. We parked up, had a bite to eat and strolled around. It's a gorgeous little town, a jewel in a pretty arid landscape. I hadn't come to Fuerteventura necessarily with a view to staying here, but to meet up with Elaine somewhere different. The place did appeal to me from the outset and we booked into a guest house for a few nights. So inevitably came the moment I stopped and looked at a little block of bright houses. Fatal attraction. I eventually tracked down the owners and spoke to the woman. Yes, there was a possibility of a let, but there was a problem. The house in question was occupied by two Belgians who had defaulted on the rent. They were presently pursuing eviction, but it might be some weeks before that would happen. In the meantime she offered to show me around another, similar house.

Well, it was perfect. Two bed, no stairs, garden, parking, with a communal swimming pool with sea water, and a small sun terrace which belonged to the house in question. Yes, I could have first refusal when and if it became available. I was delighted. Everything was starting to fall into place. I flew back to Jersey temporarily and Elaine went home to Tenerife.

After a couple more weeks back in Jersey I prepared to leave once more. I'd decided that Fuerteventura was for me. Hopefully the house in Correlejo would come my way, but my Plan B would be to find somewhere else, but there were logistics to overcome. The two cars were still in Tenerife. It was conceivable that I could drive/ferry them both over to Fuerteventura but it was a task which didn't appeal to me. I placed an advertisement in the local paper in Fuerteventura. Would someone be able to bring one of the cars over for me while I brought the other? I got a reply from Dennis. Yes, he would be happy to help me out. So, off I flew Jersey – Tenerife, Dennis flew Fuerteventura – Tenerife and we met up there. I drove my Escort and Dennis drove Richard's Renault. Off we both went, ferry to Gran Canaria, then onwards to Fuerteventura and finally the drive up to Corralejo. What a palaver, but I was getting rather used to moving everything, including myself, around like chess pieces. I stayed in an Airbnb until my house, happily, became available and I moved in.

I'm still in touch with Dennis, who's a great traveller, and who goes to see his daughter in Lanzarote often.

✈

Corralejo is one of the Canaries' most recently developed resorts, having come late to the party. Nonetheless it is now a popular spot with many expats from Italy, Britain, Ireland, Germany and elsewhere choosing to settle there. It's a fairly typical Spanish resort town with the usual bars, restaurants, shops, low-rise hotels and apartments.

It's an opportune moment, for those who don't know Spain, to mention the ubiquitous 'Chinese' shops. These are a comparatively new phenomenon, and might be likened to the Indian- and Pakistani-owned shops that sprung up in British towns and cities from the 1950s onwards. In Britain these shops catered initially to the new immigrants and made available both local and imported produce. They opened all hours, which was a shock to the sleepy and complacent British retail sector. Quickly they opened ethnic restaurants, which ironically proved way more popular with the British than with their own people. Corner shops and newsagents quickly changed hands into the ownership of those who had a fierce work ethic and a desire to better themselves.

So in Spain, the Chinese spotted a gap in the market, and not only for ethnic restaurants. There were no convenience shops where you could buy almost anything. Retail was very regimented and you needed to visit several establishments to complete your shopping. The Chinese opened premises, piled high and sold cheap, much in the manner that Marks & Spencer did originally in Britain. They sell anything, often imported goods of dubious quality, but it is a business model that works. Perhaps the modern equivalent to Pound Shops elsewhere. There are two massive Chinese shops in Corralejo.

Anyway, I settled down, started talking to people as I generally do, and met a lot of interesting people. Of course, I'd already made sure that the town was equipped with a gym, which I frequented. As night follows day, I started teaching spinning classes, my speciality, and attending yoga classes. So good was the yoga instructor Diana that I asked her if she'd teach a few classes on my sun terrace. Of course, I got my classes for free again.

I made use of my second bedroom. When I had nobody staying with me then I'd rent it out. That way the house more or less paid for itself. So I settled down once more to a simple, easy life. The more sun I got, the more I practised yoga, exercised generally, the better I felt. Still pretty constant discomfort though, and pain at times. I knew that this would always be with me but I was now more serene, coping with it. The pain no longer defined me, I was carving myself a nice life in the knowledge that my boys were both happy and successful too.

As in Tenerife, I came across a Cannabis Club. This was a more formal establishment which wasn't for any old Tom or Tomasina. When I went to enquire, they questioned me suspiciously, only softening when I persuaded them that I had no interest in smoking the stuff. I needed it purely for medicinal purposes. I had to produce medical certificates and references before I could obtain a coveted membership card. From then I was able to obtain free (free, yes I know)

cannabis oil which is simply great and useful for many medical issues including skin complaints. Other goods were discounted. There was a bar, pool table and it was only a few minutes from the house.

✈

I had a lovely lady, Lottie, visit me. We became friends and had a lot in common. She invited me to stay in Barcelona, which I did on several occasions. Her amazing apartment was in the Raval district with its fabulous vegan restaurants, bars and markets.

My friend Dawn came to visit. And this was to prove more than a fleeting visit to Fuerteventura for her.

> *Dawn says, 'I felt completely at home with Sandi in Fuerteventura. My personal issues back in Jersey seemed to melt away. Sandi somehow induces a sense of calmness, even out-of-body experiences. One day we were lying on our sunbeds and I said something like, 'I'm staying here, I'm not going back to work.' Just like that. I had the beach café at Ouaisné at the time. I rang people that I knew were interested in buying the café and we agreed a deal. Within weeks I'd bought an apartment two minutes away from Sandi's place. That's the sort of effect she has on people. I still have the apartment and go there frequently. It's my forever place'.*

José – Part 1

Along the way I'd met one or two nice men. One or two rats as well but you can't win 'em all. I was nearly 60 so neither love nor lust was uppermost in my mind. When you're a teenager, well, the opposite sex rates highly, if not top, on a girl's list of priorities. (Sometimes indeed the same sex, before I offend anyone!) At 60 it's generally slipped down the charts in favour of other things. I'd almost forgotten what it was like to be admired by a good-looking bloke! Girls, you know the way when a cute guy looks at you that way, maybe says 'Hi!' and you know that way that your face goes hot, you unconsciously brush back your hair with your fingers, push back your shoulders and say 'Hi!' back, body language all positive? Well, that was the day I met José.

Dawn and I were at the beach and this good looking, long, dark curly-haired and bronzed fit Spanish body caught my eye. We started chatting and flirting. A fun afternoon. A simple guy, as in easy going. We shared fruit and chatted, although his English was a little mixed up but understandable.

I arranged to meet up with him the next afternoon. I liked the fact that he was into healthy eating, exercise and a non-drinker, although he did roll his own fags. Dawn was staying with me at the time and he came back for a drink. He only drank water, no tea or coffee. We all sat in the garden and enjoyed the sunshine. I was a little nervous as I think he wanted sex. Finally I said to Dawn that I couldn't do it. It had been such a long time, since before my accident 12 years previously. OMG was it that long? Here I was at 60 contemplating having sex with a younger guy. 12 years younger, but I guess these days that's not so much. Dawn said 'Oh just go for it. It may wake you up.' Well it certainly did. I lost lots of weight and felt amazing.

Richard, Laura, André and Debs all met José and didn't disapprove. They didn't exactly approve either – maybe they sensed something that I didn't. Anyway, they were a great few months but I ought to have known it wouldn't last forever. Newlyweds really mean it when they make their vows but lust rarely runs smoothly.

I invited José to officially move in. That was the worst thing that I could have done, though in my defence, I couldn't have foreseen it. He became controlling, not outrageously at first, just little things. The way he spoke. 'Where are you going? How long will you be?' It had been many years since I'd been answerable to anybody and it made me uncomfortable. I thought maybe I ought to give him some leeway, a bit of give and take.

Then came my 60th birthday party which took place in my house. Dawn had persuaded me to have one, and she arranged it. She invited loads of people, some of whom I didn't know – well maybe I'd met them once or something. There were men, other men, all of whom José glowered at and refused to talk to. Like they were all planning to kidnap me and make off into the night. It was a side of him that I didn't like.

Meanwhile I continued to flit back and forth to Jersey. Jersey has always been my home base. José stayed in the house if I happened to be away. Things continued to unravel. It was a few months before my lease was up and I had every intention of renewing it. Then the owners turned up next door, out of the blue, on holiday. It just didn't feel right. (As I may have mentioned before, I think I have a bit of intuition at times, what the Irish sometimes call 'the Sight'. Again, it must be through my mother's Irish genes. A bit of healing power too, though much good that has done me personally.)

Another odd thing happened. The lady owner knocked at my door one day and asked if they could keep a box of stuff on my roof terrace. I didn't get a straight answer when I asked why, or what. Then one day the owners' agent arrived, struggling under the weight of the 'box' in question. I protested but he said that he had his orders (or whatever the Spanish equivalent is). It felt all wrong. I became sure that the lease wasn't going to be renewed, but I didn't ask, which I probably ought to have done.

I'd had enough of José complicating my life. I told him he'd have to leave – the lease was running out so he couldn't stay. He begged for time, he cried right in front of me clasping his hands. I was about to leave for a few days in Jersey and so I relented. He could stay for now but he was starting to wear me out.

I returned to Corralejo a week later. There was a bracelet on my bedroom floor. It wasn't mine. José was watching TV. 'Whose is this bracelet?' I asked.
'No idea, isn't it yours?' he shrugged.
Maybe I was going mad. Maybe it was my bracelet and I hadn't recognised it. I said nothing more but my instincts

were on high alert. Two days later I got a call from a woman. It went something like this.

'Hello, is that Sandi?'

'Yes that's me.'

'Oh hello Sandi. My name's Sofia. I'm José's ex-girlfriend. I thought I had to speak to you.'

'Oh?'

'Look, this is difficult but I think you need to know. José's not a nice man. He's a pig.'

'Er well...'

'The thing is, I know he's your boyfriend now but...'

'But?'

'I sort of slept with him, in your bed, while you were away. I thought you ought to know. I'm sorry.'

'Oh. Have you lost a bracelet by any chance?'

'I wondered where that was.'

'Maybe I can hand it back to you. Fancy coffee sometime?'

I was quite calm. My intuition was proving correct. After talking with Sofia I went into the lounge and told him to pack and leave right now. He was in shock and started crying. 'Just pack up and go now,' I insisted.

He left, but next morning he was on my doorstep again. 'Please give me another chance.' That's exactly what he was, a 'chancer'. I considered the matter and let him back on my terms, as a lodger, no further relationship. He accepted that. He had previously lived with his yoga teacher friend Joan (male, pronounced Joanne), but his father had arrived from Almeria to stay for a while. Joan had a little boy to care for when he wasn't with his mother, although

José would childmind for Joan when he was teaching. There was now no room for José to live with Joan.

When José finally left the house, he went to live in Joan's ex-wife's boat in the harbour. I think he's still there.

A Curiosity

Back in 1956, the year that I was born, if you had a half crown you were rich. Even a shilling would get you into the Saturday morning matinée at the local cinema, a bag of sweets to break your teeth on, and a penny or two left over. But if an auntie were to give you a half crown for your birthday, or if you maybe found one in the street, then you'd hide it away, dreaming of all the things you might buy, the places you could go.

So imagine my delight when, weeding and trowelling in my little garden in Correlejo one day, that's exactly what I found. A perfect British half crown, dated 1956, the year of my birth. What were the chances, and how had it come to be there? I'll never know, but these sorts of things seem to follow me around.

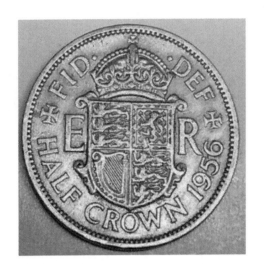

Biking

My sporting days had long gone. I was just physically unable to jog, with the impact and stress throughout the body that this involves. Rowing was completely out of the question, but I remembered the satisfaction, the buzz, that strenuous activity induced. I was able to replicate that feeling to a degree with spinning, but cycling in the outdoors brings scenery, the wind in your face, the sense of freedom. Now and again Dawn and I would hop on the ferry to Lanzarote. It is no distance from Corralejo and the terrain is more inviting to the casual biker. That's not to say that there aren't challenging climbs for those (like my son) who seek them out. We'd generally skirt the foothills of the volcanic Ajaches, admiring them rather than taking them on. Frequent stops, a spot of lunch, a bit of shopping back in Playa Blanca before catching the ferry home.

Richard brought me an electric bike over. In fact he brought two. One was for Tess, my partner in our former business of wholesale florist suppliers in Jersey. Tess's brother Mike had also bought a property in Corralejo. She came regularly and stayed at Mike's beautiful house right on the beach. Dawn and I would get invites to lunch, sitting by the pool.

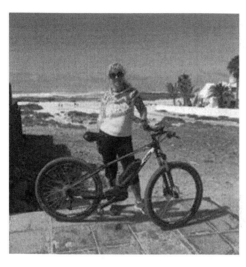

My electric bike - note thick tyres for the terrain

Ayahuasca

It was around this time that a girl came to lodge with me. Inviting tourists to stay, you never know really what sort of people are going to turn up, despite the pre-booking checks. Anyway this girl was lovely, but also unconventional. She was into herbal medicine, potions and the rest. We had some interesting chats.

She started talking about ayahuasca. 'What now?' I hear you cry. Ok, it's a psychoactive substance made out of certain vine leaves and other ingredients found in the Amazon. It is mashed and boiled to make a brew. It is traditionally used by indigenous people such as the tribes of the Peruvian Amazon. Along with psychological stress and psychedelic effects on the mind, it is said to have medicinal purging properties. The usual advice is to take ayahuasca only under the guidance of a trained shaman.

Spiritual awakening has been claimed by non-traditional users. As I am certain that I had my own spiritual awakening after my accident I was all ears. I was feeling troubled by José at the time. Maybe I could purge him away? Maybe this wonderful stuff had a pain relief element. I was intrigued, but hesitant to head off to the Amazon. A bit of research led to the happy discovery that there was an ayahuasca weekend centre just a 45-minute flight away, in Tegueste, north Tenerife. A three-day programme. Before I knew what I was doing, I was booked up. Dawn thought I was mad.

Things started inauspiciously. It was cold in north Tenerife, high up in the mountains. I hadn't brought enough clothes. I got lost. Eventually I found Tegueste which is only a few kilometres from the airport but in the middle of nowhere. Eliel, the facilitator of the programme, came and found me and took me to the lodge which housed the retreat centre. It was very simple, as I'd expected, something like a hostel. They served vegetarian food, again simple but wholesome. I was a bit surprised to find that there were as many as 20 guests. They were from all over the world. That being the case I imagined that many were returners and that the place had earned itself a good reputation. Still, I was apprehensive and didn't really know what to expect.

I had an initial chat with Eliel, and I tried to explain why I was there. I'd decided my prime wish was to be rid of José though I didn't quite know how to accomplish this. Eliel assured me that, after three days at the retreat, I would be on the way to releasing him. Then he offered me a choice of sleeping arrangements. I could sleep in the big room with everyone else, or I could have a private room all to myself. Well, it was no contest. I wasn't going to muck in with everyone else, I'd go private, thank you very much. Then, the first of many strange things happened. When I saw everyone together in the big room, I changed my mind. I wanted to be with them. I wanted to be part of the shared experience throughout the night.

There was a group introductory session in which everyone participated. Eliel explained in detail how the ceremony worked, what was done, what may happen. He assured us that things *would* indeed happen. We might become scared but we would be looked after, we were in a safe place.

So we settled down. We each had our sleeping bag, pillow, blanket, bucket. Bucket? Ah yes, this was for the purging. We might, probably would, be throwing up in the course of the night. Maybe worse, as I'd read and been told.

Then the Shaman, Elian, came in, the first time we'd seen him. Well he was tall, blond, handsome like an old-fashioned film star. There was something else about him – magnetic, compelling, captivating, beautiful. I couldn't take my eyes off him. He spoke a few words before disappearing again. Then the music began, medicine music we called it. Pipes, flutes, all redolent of the Amazon. Some people started dancing, others swaying, yet others like me sat there enjoying the music, the experience. In truth it was getting past my bedtime and I needed my sleep. I was told not to worry, I'd get my sleep all right.

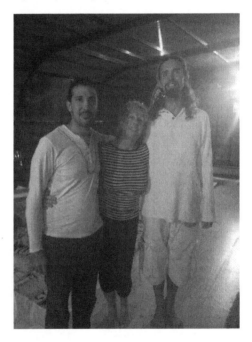

Eliel, Sandi & Elian (Shaman)

Now the Shaman, Elian, reappeared. He'd been preparing the ayahuasca. The leaves are mashed and boiled, much as I did with my cannabis plants. It produces a vile brew. The Shaman came to each of us in turn and offered us this stuff. Having paid for the programme, you're hardly likely to turn it down. However he suggested, and I agreed, that as a first-timer it would be better to have a smaller portion to begin with. He performed his ritual and urged me now to think of the thing or things I wanted to be rid of. I thought of José and how I wished to cast him aside. Then he fed me the ayahuasca. Ugh, it tasted dreadful. The music continued, more softly now. Everyone lay down quietly.

It took about two hours. Then a guy started screaming (it turned out he'd recently lost his brother). A girl next to me started sobbing her heart out. Others reacted in different ways – talking, shouting, crying. Several were sick into their buckets. None of this worried me, it was expected and seemed natural. Eliel and Elian visited each of us in turn, talking, comforting. They came to me. I started telling them about José, but then, without warning, I threw up into the bucket. It was the purging of the toxins, of José. Then, gentle reader, to my horror I pooed my pants! They understood and took me to the loo where I changed, and I was none the worse. Returning to my place, I lay down listening to the gentle music. I was at peace. I fell asleep.

The second day and night followed a similar pattern, fortunately less the inadvertent pooing. By day we ate the lovely veggie food. We walked in the nearby mountains of Tegueste. We slept, to make up for that which we had lost the previous night. On the second night, after the taking of the ayahuasca, I started chatting – to Eliel, the Shaman, anyone who would listen. This time, thoughts of my sons surfaced, I needed to voice them. I was worried about Richard. Why was he conforming, going against his free spirit? I didn't understand until a few months later when he split up with his long-time girlfriend. She was so lovely, but I guess that Rich, like me, needed to move on. I wasn't so concerned about André. To an outsider I might have sounded like a bar room drunk. But here, in this environment, everything seemed normal and natural. Everyone had their own experiences and manifested them in different ways.

By the third and final night I'd done my purging. Now it was just euphoria. I danced with the beautiful Shaman. Everything was perfect. I had reached some sort of nirvana and wanted to stay forever.

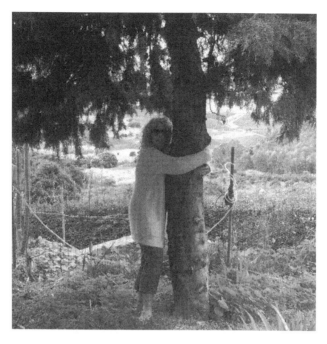

Tree hug, Ayahuasca ceremony

Ibiza

During this latter part of my life in Fuerteventura I was spending a lot of time away. José looked after the guests. By this time I was determined to leave the island. It seemed to be the only way that I was to be finally rid of him. Despite all its wonders, the ayahuasca had not magically disappeared him. Now I was back in Jersey for a few days. I bought a camper van. On a whim. Don't ask me why. As I've mentioned, my life now seemed to consist of snap decisions. Not all of those decisions were wise, but in this, my Life#2, it seemed to be important to me to make them,

164

for better or worse, rather than waste time dithering. Anyway, blame Richard. He encouraged me to go ahead and buy it if I wanted. So I did, immediately customising it with colourful flower decals. It was like something from the Summer of Love (1967 to you young ones, flower power, free love, hippies and all that). It was certainly distinctive.

I was scared to drive the thing, but now I just had to get on with it. By this time, I was running out of islands but I had a fancy to go to Ibiza, one island south of Mallorca and well known to young British visitors in particular. One of my ex-partners in my wholesale florist days was Tess. She agreed to come along. So off we set, yet again – France, Spain, ferry from Barcelona to Ibiza.

I wasn't entirely struck on Ibiza really. We stayed a few days there, had a look around. Then Tess decided that she'd seen enough. She flew back home, leaving me on my own. I'm normally fine with my own company but I didn't feel at ease in Ibiza in the camper really. But, as always, I got chatting to people. In particular I got chatting to a girl, Petra. She was fine and we became quite friendly. We got talking about accommodation. Now Ibiza isn't the cheapest place I've visited and inevitably, it seemed, we started discussing the possibility of sharing an apartment, to cut costs. As I said, I wasn't particularly sold on Ibiza but I didn't particularly want to go back to Fuerteventura where I'd need to confront José again, and where my lease was due to run out anyway. In the end I decided to head back, but promised that, if Petra found a suitable two-bed apartment in Ibiza, to get in touch. I also left the camper van there with a lot of my stuff.

Back in Corralejo, José was as polite and subservient as before, so I decided against a further confrontation. I couldn't face it anyway. Soon enough came the call from Ibiza. Petra had found the perfect apartment. She needed to pay the deposit and of course I made a payment to her for my share. Back I went to Ibiza, though not without José plaintively hinting that he ought to come too.

Going to Ibiza was a big mistake. Everything had changed. I'd told Petra when I'd be arriving and, though she may or may not have said so, I assumed that she'd be there at the airport to meet me. I gave her the benefit of the doubt as I'd left the camper van nearby. I called her, got directions, and eventually I got to the 'perfect' new apartment under my own steam.

I wished I hadn't. I was greeted coldly, completely different from the old Petra though I couldn't understand why. I knew she liked a bit of a drink so maybe that was something to do with it. As to the apartment, well, she had more or less claimed it for herself, maybe choosing to forget that we'd agreed to share equally. The bigger of the two bedrooms she had claimed for herself leaving me with a small, shabby room and a cheap bed which smelled of cat's pee. The living and kitchen areas were strewn with her own bags and boxes. My reasonable protests had no effect. Clearly she thought that I'd shrug my shoulders and accept the situation. Either that or she was so stupid that she couldn't see that the whole thing was rigged in her favour. I was speechless as she turned on the television, ignoring me.

Without another word I left. Stunned, I wandered down a street or two before sitting down in a coffee shop for a water and a think. It didn't take long for me to realise I'd made a bad decision. I waited until the coast was clear, retrieved the bag I'd left in the apartment, jumped in the camper van and high-tailed it back to the airport and, eventually, Fuerteventura. Petra harassed me in the days that followed, wanting to know what was wrong, demanding I keep my promise. In the end I just ignored her. Sod my share of the advance rental I owed; she could sing for it.

Dawn says, 'I had family staying in my own apartment nearby, so I was squatting with José at Sandi's place. I got along okay with José, he's a nice bloke. But at that time Sandi was providing and José was taking. It seemed to me to be a sort-of one-way thing. When José got jealous, it was because he feared Sandi would no longer be at his beck and call.

'Me and Sandi are alike in that we both love the sunshine and we get a bit gloomy in Jersey when it gets cold and miserable. I admire Sandi so much for reaching out for travel and adventures, following her instincts. No one would have blamed her for feeling sorry for herself after that terrible accident. She's inspiring.

'Sandi does doubt herself at times, but goes ahead and acts anyway. It usually comes good. She makes her own luck. And she has this ability of getting others to do things.

I still have my place in Fuerteventura though Sandi's no longer there. But my life has been much better for knowing her.'

Mallorca again

*What a wonderful way to live
She's travelling all over the world
Why, the fame and all the opportunities unfurled
(Sandy Denny)*

I sat in the ferry queue at Puerto del Rosario, Cadiz-bound. Also in the queue, right next to me, was a large black car, Mafia-type, with driver, wife and child. I thought nothing more of it until later when we'd set sail. I bumped into the driver on deck and we got chatting (his family had left the car before boarding). Small world. It transpired that he was the main supplier for the Cannabis Club in Corralejo! If ever I was to go back to Fuerteventura I was to contact him for the best deals. Though how he could do better deals than the ones I had been getting I really don't know.

We arrived in Cadiz after what is a long journey, two nights on a freighter. I drove away with no particular destination in mind. I wasn't that bothered really. My long-term plan was to head back to Jersey but I could take my time. I headed north-east to Granada and, getting into tourist mode, booked a few nights in a hotel there. Everywhere was cheaper right now, being out of season. Indeed the snow was on the mountain tops. Granada is lovely. The buildings have an intriguing mix of Islamic, Moorish and Spanish about them. Some of the buildings and monuments are wonderful, as are the plentiful parks and gardens. It was certainly chilly though and that is something my body just doesn't appreciate or desire.

So where could I go to get a bit of sunshine? I remembered José and Joan telling me that Almeria was the best place in mainland Spain for sunshine. That wasn't so far away, back down to the south coast, so off I set. Almeria is a beautiful city all right with its Moorish influences, civil war tunnels and free tapas. Again, it didn't call to me to stay longer.

I drove slowly northwards, along the coastline – Cartagena, Alicante, Benidorm. By this time I was getting quite concerned about my trusty Escort. I'd looked after it, ensured it got serviced regularly, but it was by now 24 years old. It still seemed to be running sweetly however and I took a fatalistic attitude. Whatever would be would be. Then I came to Denia on the Costa Blanca. Denia's a lovely little port town. It's been happily overlooked to an extent by the masses and therefore retains an authentic Spanish vibe. I'll go back one day, but now I heard the Balearics calling to me again. As I'd got closer to Denia the more aware I became that it had ferry links to the islands. Should I head out that way again, completing the circle? I had no other firm plans.

I drove down to the harbour area, parked up and found the ferry office. Any sailings to Mallorca perhaps? A tentative enquiry. 'Si señora, en una hora.' In an hour! Destiny was calling, there was no doubt about it. I booked a ticket and was on my way. I had nowhere to stay when I got there, but I've never had a problem with finding temporary digs. A single middle-aged woman is welcome most anywhere; easily pleased and unlikely to be much bother. Nonetheless I made a call or two on the ferry. I knew a lady called Sandra from my previous time in Mallorca who owned a couple of apartments in the north of the island. Yes, she said, of course I could stay in one of her apartments. Only for a couple of months though as she would be letting it out at tourist rates when the season kicked in. That was fine by me. I wasn't looking to settle permanently.

So we docked at Palma, I coaxed the Escort into life once more and headed north for Puerto Pollensa, about 55 kilometres away where I met Sandra. The apartment was just right and I settled in happily. The town is small enough, about six kilometres from Pollensa town itself. It is quiet but with lovely walks and an interesting town centre. Most importantly, it was virtually on the fabulous beach area. As I've mentioned, I find sea bathing so beneficial. I imagine it all goes back to my aqua therapy days when the feeling of weightlessness brought profound pain relief. When I'm paddling around in the warm sea water it is blissful.

Also essentially, there was a gym. It was a 20-minute walk away but I'd head there most days for a gentle workout and to participate in yoga and spinning classes. As always, I also met some nice people to talk to – I was certainly never lonely. All in all, it was a pleasant time.

The time came when Sandra needed the apartment back, though I guess I might have stayed if I'd been willing to pay the tourist rate. A small concern then, I had to start flat hunting. The concern lasted only a very short time. Within minutes of stepping through the door of an estate agent I'd been offered a 2-bed apartment nearby, at a reasonable rent. I took it there and then. Of course, I didn't need two bedrooms, but I reckoned I could always get someone to share if needs be. Anyway, I'd been talking to my friend Janet in Birmingham. Eventually it was agreed that she'd come over to stay, and that was what happened. For several months we shared the apartment. We mostly did our own separate thing though Janet happily came along with me to yoga classes. It was a nice time.

I found the local Cannabis Club! I was getting an old hand at this. Danny and his girlfriend Grace, an English couple ran it, calling it the Ovni Club. It was no easy matter finding it, or being admitted, but once it was accepted that I had genuine medical reasons it was fine and they were as good as gold, and incredibly helpful. Which was just as well as I was soon to be troubled by another health scare. It started off as a bit of a rash across my chest. I took no notice really, rubbed on a bit of cream, but it steadily got worse, and pretty unsightly. I went to the doctor who prescribed stronger cream. It had no effect. He referred me to the hospital in the town of Inca, which was a few miles away. They told me that the lumps (no longer just a rash) would need to be cut out and could indeed be cancerous.

That scared me. I showed Danny my chest at the Cannabis Club. No problem, they would give me something. They did just that, a powerful mixture which I was warned to be very careful with, to be applied externally. I was told not to make any plans to do anything else after using it. So, for a month, I applied this stuff religiously and hoped. I was high as a kite most of the time, only emerging from the apartment occasionally, like a mole, when the effects had died down a little. I had been told to check out of normal life for a month. I reckoned that would have been the case at the hospital anyway, so that wasn't a concern. Getting better was.

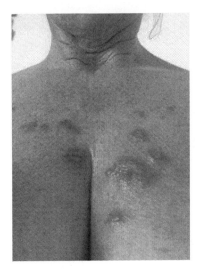

I got better. The lumps and bumps slowly subsided. Today you can hardly see a mark. Yet the mainline medical profession refuse to have anything to do with this sort of treatment which gets results. Medical cannabis has a long and successful history. Pain relief is one of the most common uses. It is only in more modern times, as governments have brought in a myriad of regulations to control medical prescriptions, that cannabis has been side-lined as 'unsafe'. Where it is allowed in certain limited circumstances, doctors are still reluctant to prescribe. This allows Big Pharma to continue controlling their markets and maximising profits, and it's why a readily available and proven substance is regarded as the Devil's work.

Danny and Grace at the Ovni Club were incredibly kind and helpful to me. The club was raided a few years ago and harshly closed down for a time. Grace was expecting at the time. She's since had a baby boy and they live in a lovely country villa in Mallorca.

✈

Eventually, both me and Janet were ready to move on. In any case, this had always been a stepping stone for Janet. She has a son in New Zealand and eventually left to stay with him. I believe she's still there.

'What about your camper van?' I hear you cry. That's right. It was still in Ibiza, safely locked up. As my time in Mallorca was coming to an end, I went and brought it back, so I now had two vehicles sitting in Puerto Pollensa. I had intended to sell the camper van at this stage, but as it transpired, it still had a part to play in my life.

I was inclined to head back to Jersey for a while. Maybe my wandering days were over, for now at least. I'd never really left Jersey in my own mind, but had just taken breaks away from the island. Like so many people that have arrived in Jersey never intending to stay, that island has eventually become a permanent home. During my Spanish island hopping I'd often made quick trips back to Jersey. Air travel had become like taking a bus for me, quite routine and a non-event.

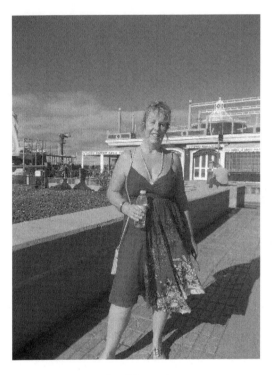

Sandi in purple

So I had both the Escort and the camper van. Now fate intervened so that I was left with only the one. I'd recently had the Escort fully serviced. It was 24 years old and had served me faithfully. Only fairly recently I'd had it fitted with a new sun roof. I was headed to Palma airport to catch a flight back to Jersey, intending to leave the car at the airport. For some reason I set out for the airport early. It was no more than an hour's drive but something made me set off with several hours to spare. Half way through my journey, smoke started pouring out of the bonnet. Alarmed,

I pulled over. The water gauge was in the red. I jumped out, bewildered. There I was, stranded.

I managed to call my insurance company and a garage. Along came a tow truck to take it away. It transpired that the one thing that the service centre had not done was to top up the coolant. It was repairable, but the garage said that really it was not economical. The sell-on value of the car was low, primarily due to its age. It was probably only worth repairing for my own sentimental value, otherwise the sensible thing would be to scrap it. I took the sensible course of action and waved my faithful friend goodbye. The garage said that they would scrap it for free as they could use the relatively new tyres and other bits and pieces. They also paid for a taxi so I could get to the airport.

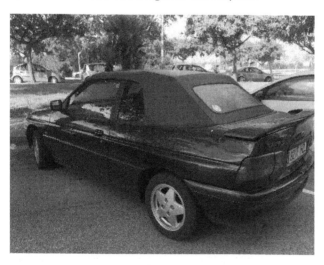

Some time later I got a certificate of scrappage from them. To me it felt like a death certificate. This amazing car looked after me so well during my travels. These days I don't even own a vehicle, just an amazing e-bike.

Later I returned to Puerto Pollensa and loaded up the camper van with my remaining possessions. I'd decided to return to Jersey for a while. This time I'd decided to travel by ferry to Toulon. From there I spent a little time with a friend, Sophie Denis, in Cannes. Sophie is French and originally from Lyon. She's a clairvoyant and I'd first met her a few years previously in Mallorca. I decided to stay with her and her two girls for a few days. Her husband had left her for a younger model. It was great catching up, and of course she read my cards. Apparently, I was to meet my soulmate in a year or two! (Still waiting.) We went to see her mother who lives in the hills, and we swam in the amazing infinity pool overlooking Cannes.

From Cannes I then headed north for St Malo. I did the long drive non-stop but arrived in St Malo just too late for the evening sailing to Jersey. Happily, I was able to sleep in the camper van before getting the morning sailing.

I stayed with Richard and sold the camper van within two days, getting my money back. It was July 2017.

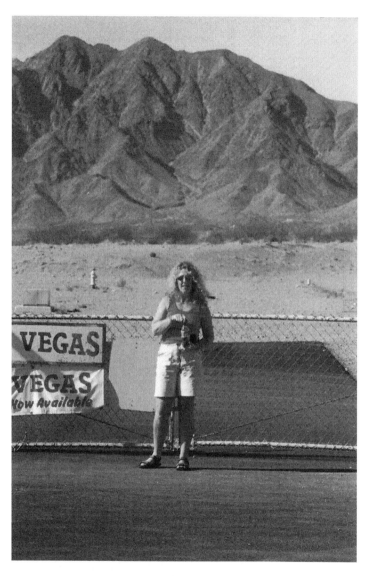

Sandi in Vegas

Jersey

Beautiful Jersey, gem of the sea
Ever my heart turns in longing to thee
Bright are the mem'ries you waken for me
Beautiful Jersey, gem of the sea

So I was back home, back to base camp as it were. Richard and Katie, together with little Beth, had bought a nice house in St Martin. They had a spare room and were happy to offer it to me. And, to be honest, I wanted to settle down for a little while now. My health wasn't the best and my frequent travelling and moving had probably left me a little run down. This in addition to the aches and pains resulting from my accident from which I relentlessly sought relief.

Some while back I had spent five days in hospital in Tenerife with suspected appendicitis. They had fed me antibiotics and let me go. I'd try to ignore that problem, I had plenty of others. It came back to bite. I was feeling particularly tired and ill one day, so much so that Richard insisted I get myself checked out at the General Hospital. This I did, and was immediately admitted and the offending appendix removed. The staff at the hospital expressed amazement that I had continued with the condition for so long. The operation had an unfortunate side-effect in opening up a hernia at the point of incision, another thing I have only recently had fixed.

I started having dizzy spells, vertigo. Often I'd wake in the early hours feeling most peculiar, and quite ill. On several occasions I was so concerned that I called for an ambulance – I was getting to be quite a loyal customer down at A&E. They ran tests. All they could find was low blood pressure, hypotension. As you know, I'm not a fan of conventional drugs. There are ways of dealing with hypotension and I do my best. Adding salt to my diet seems to help.

I was constantly assessing my future. Should I go abroad again, especially as the Jersey winter was about to set in? My health issues, plus financial constraints, led me to believe that Jersey was the best place for me right now. I was conscious that I was a non-paying guest in someone else's house and, when the day came that Richard gently asked me how long I was going to stay, I had to take action. I needed to acquire a place of my own. I visited a couple of estate agents – I'd worked in the business years ago so I was recognised. Jersey isn't the easiest place to find affordable accommodation, but I was tentatively shown a basement flat in the north of St Helier. It was a tip, thanks to the previous tenants, but I was able to see through the mess. The owner was happy to let to me, though it was agreed that new carpet and a paint job were necessary beforehand.

I was delighted, and of course Richard and Katie were pleased at the prospect of having their house back to themselves. When I finally took possession, the place was unfurnished. I placed an ad in the 'Wanted' section of the Jersey Evening Post. I was soon fighting off people wanting to offload their furniture and stuff, and I took the best of it. So, as at February 2020 I have a small flat in a Victorian terrace in a quiet road on the northern fringe of St Helier. It has several rooms which I've decorated fancifully, as you can imagine. I have a yoga room where I hold classes. In future these will include yoga and meditation for those in addiction recovery, and perhaps 'accessible' yoga for those with physical limitations. I continue to teach spinning classes at a local gym, where my old, trusty 70s/80s soundtracks continue to be well received as a counterpoint to the more modern music generally in vogue elsewhere.

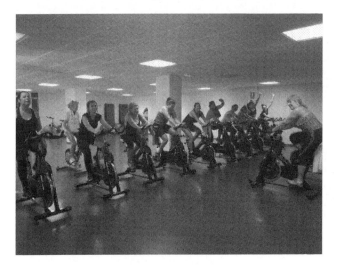

Feel Fit Gym, Corralejo

I'm blessed to have had that spiritual awakening after that catastrophic fall back in 2005. I'm blessed to have such great sons and so many supportive friends. I've led a life that I would never have envisaged before that fateful night, a life that was going nowhere.

Much earlier in this book I said that I lived in my head for years rather than my heart. Today I live with my emotional feelings very differently, and sometimes not easily, but yoga and meditation help me these days. I also believe in a higher power, a god, spiritual power, call it what you wish, looking over me.

I loved the feeling of flannelette sheets on my bed as a child. I still do!

André and his future wife Debs were living in Christchurch, New Zealand and lived through earthquakes in 2009, 2010 and 2011.

He says 'The quake struck at 12.51pm on February 22. I was working in an office in Christchurch city centre – it started to disintegrate around us, and we got out fast. 50 metres away the CTV building collapsed, killing 115 people. I had to get across town to Debbie and our home in New Brighton. It was chaos of course, a nightmare. Dead bodies, people screaming. It took me four hours. Amazingly our house was still standing, many weren't.

'We went north for a few days for respite. There's no doubt the quakes affected us mentally and ultimately it was the catalyst for us leaving New Zealand, or we might still be there.'

Today André and Debs live in Cornwall with my three beautiful granddaughters Evie, Arianna and Amaiya. When time allows, Debs practises as an acupuncturist.

André maintains that he's not at all sure what he does for a living! He has developed his love of sport and fitness and now teaches body combat, group fitness, exercise to music and spinning.

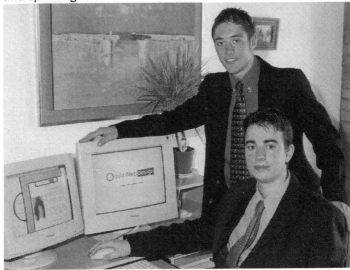

André (standing) with Andy Begeman

Richard is now in his prime as a sportsman, still cycling of course but now with triathlon as his main focus. He is part-owner of Big Maggy's, a shop which offers elite cycling products, services and accessories and which incorporates a coffee and sandwiches concession. It is situated in the heart of St Helier's finance centre. He lives in Jersey with his partner Katie and her daughter Beth.

> *Remember Terri from earlier? She says, 'Over the years Sandra and I frequently met. She was a dear friend to have and a shoulder to lean on. I was extremely proud to be asked to be her bridesmaid at her and Dick's wedding. I left the Island in December 1982, but thankfully we kept in touch.*
>
> *'Later I would return to the Island every other year with my husband and children and we all would meet up and our kids would have fun together. Her two boys are a credit to her.*
>
> *'I was very shocked and worried when I heard Sandra had fallen downstairs and broken her neck. I worried how would she manage and would she be okay, but in Sandra style she battled on and came out the other side.*
>
> *'Thankfully we have kept in touch over the years. I have loved hearing about her travels and change in career paths through social media. Her special moments of becoming a Yaya (grandmother in Spanish) and celebrating the achievements of her boys.*
>
> *I now live with my husband in York.'*

✈

Elaine? She still lives in Tenerife with her husband, still working with holistic therapies. She is in the process of opening a charity shop, Care4Cats.

✈

Joyce is a devoted wife and mother with three wonderful children. She has a lovely home in St Clement here in Jersey and we see each other quite often.

Rachel has been married to Ray for many years. Having partnered Ray in business until his recent retirement she now keeps her hand in with seasonal work. They have four grown-up children: Hannah, Lorna, James and Robert. Rachel and Ray now have the time to travel and see them all. For many years Rachel coached track and field at Jersey Spartans.

✈

Three years ago Rachel suggested I join a House and Animal Sitting site – her friend's daughter travels around the world doing this, paying only small expenses. I joined, and my first 'sit' was in Dubai in a beautiful house in a gated area with private pool, for two Saluki dogs. I was only three hours away from India, thinking 'Should I?' There followed two more sits, in Malaga and Sweden, visiting Copenhagen on the way.

A Yin Yoga Teachers' Training Course came up in Goa. I checked it out and decided to go. It was 100 hours training over two weeks. Now, back in Jersey, I have been practising and teaching Yin Yoga. Sometimes I don't feel good enough but my students tell me different. Then I decided to take another course in Gibraltar, Teacher Training for Accessible Yoga teaching people with disabilities or limited mobility. I wonder where this will lead, or take me next?

I can't wait. Life is a journey. Let's go and enjoy our time on this planet, wherever that may be.

I would recommend that everyone writes an autobiography. It has been a healing and therapeutic experience – better than any therapist!

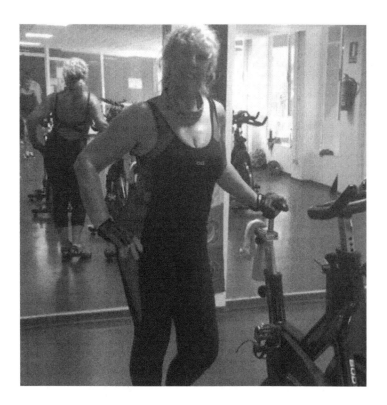

Printed in Great Britain
by Amazon